MORE FROM THE GLUTEN-FREE GOURMET

BETTE HAGMAN

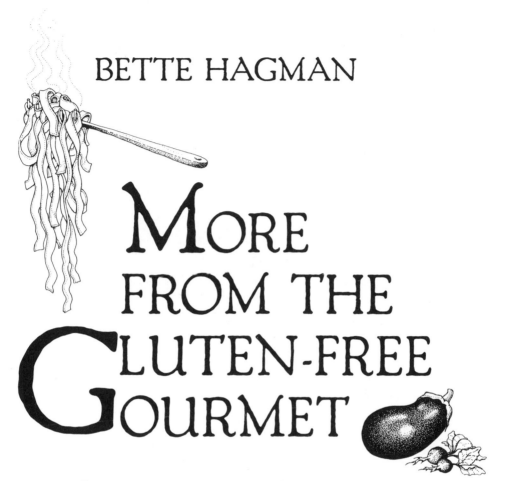

MORE FROM THE GLUTEN-FREE GOURMET

Delicious Dining Without Wheat

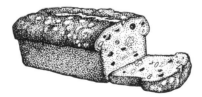

AN OWL BOOK
HENRY HOLT AND COMPANY
NEW YORK

Henry Holt and Company, LLC
Publishers since 1866
115 West 18th Street
New York, New York 10011

Henry Holt® is a registered trademark
of Henry Holt and Company, LLC.

Distributed in Canada by H. B. Fenn and Company Ltd.

Grateful acknowledgment is made to Bonnie S. Mickelson
for the corn soup recipe (Fresh Corn Chowder) from her book
Hollyhocks and Radishes (Pickle Point Publishing, Bellevue,
Wash., 1989) copyright © 1989 by Bonnie S. Mickelson.

Library of Congress Cataloging-in-Publication Data
Hagman, Bette.—Rev. ed.
More from the gluten-free gourmet : delicious
dining without wheat / Bette Hagman.
p. cm.
ISBN 0-8050-6524-5
1. Gluten-free diet—Recipes. 2. Wheat-free
diet—Recipes. I. Title.
RM237.86.H34 1993   92-30281
641.5'631—dc20   CIP

Henry Holt books are available for special promotions and
premiums. For details contact: Director, Special Markets.

First published in hardcover in 1993 by
Henry Holt and Company

First Owl Books Edition 1994

Illustrations by Laura Hartman

Printed in the United States of America

3 5 7 9 10 8 6 4

This book is dedicated to Mary Gunn,
who kept me cooking, and to the many others
who give generously of time and
talent to help fellow celiacs
find good health.

CONTENTS

PREFACE

When I finished writing *The Gluten-free Gourmet* I figured I'd included enough recipes to keep any celiac or wheat-allergic person
eating happily into the next century. I'd given recipes for pizza, pasta,
bread, and desserts. What more could one desire?

The answer seems to be *more* of the same. By the time my first
cookbook went into publication, I was already back at the stove
working out new recipes. And, as soon as the book came out in print,
your letters told me you felt as I did. Let's have *more*.

I definitely wasn't a cook when I started; I still think of myself as
more of an experimenter challenged by the diet. Before my diagnosis,
that had created a dilemma—should I eat and suffer afterward or
abstain and continue to lose weight? But, with the elimination of
gluten, I have found a new pleasure in eating.

I first planned this second book to be a collection of exotic foreign
flavors, the idea germinating when I realized that I didn't dare taste
any of those delicious-looking, wonderful-smelling mixed dishes
served on my travels. (It's practically impossible to translate *toxic
glutens* into a language one doesn't speak.) With the help of cookbooks and three cooking teachers who specialize in foreign dishes, I
worked out gluten-free adaptations for some of those recipes. But
those were only the beginning of this book.

Some of the recipes in this volume are my choice; but *more* of the
book is yours. Readers have told me what they want—more breads,
more desserts, and more casseroles—and many sent along recipes
they had developed. I listened and cooked. I'd work out a recipe in

my kitchen and then my testers—twenty in all, across the United States—cooked, corrected, altered, and fed their families from the recipes I sent them. I've received feedback ranging from "Wonderful! When am I going to be able to share this recipe?" to "My kids wouldn't touch it. They said it looked like green slime."

The final impetus for *More* came from the growing popularity of the automated bread makers. Since machines and I have the same affinity for one another as a bare foot for a bent pin in the carpet, I delayed purchasing one until shamed into it. I immediately wondered why I had waited. Breads now take five minutes of my time instead of the former four and one-half hours, and I am able to experiment without pain, perfecting a wide range of new recipes.

This book is not planned to be a gluten-free diet book. We can find plenty of nutritious food within our safe diet list, but the thought of a lifetime of simply cooked foods can lead to boredom in eating (and to cheating). Here I've concentrated on dishes to enhance, at times, the simple foods on the diet, and even more important, to save work for the cook, who can now feed the whole family great-tasting dishes without having to create a separate meal for the dieter.

As in *The Gluten-free Gourmet*, I included scores of exciting recipes for breads, pastries, cakes, cookies, and desserts, and since these are the first cravings for those who have to live on a wheat-free or gluten-free diet (and the hardest to find commercially made), these sections are placed first in this cookbook. I've also added in the following sections new recipes for chicken, meat, seafood, and vegetable dishes, many of them casseroles, which we have to avoid eating in restaurants. I gave recipes for various pastas and four pizza crusts in my first book, so, to avoid duplication in this volume, I have included pastas only in casseroles and have suggested just one bread recipe that makes a good pizza crust. I have created six convenient dry mixes that one can use at home or carry on trips (see page 329).

Again, I have used eggs and milk (or cream) and butter generously in many recipes, but, because many celiacs are lactose intolerant, especially when first diagnosed, I have suggested alternatives for them in every recipe possible. (See page 17, "Cooking with Gluten-free Flours and Other Substitutes," for substitutes for dairy products, soy, corn, and eggs and suggestions for other dietary problems.)

To make the recipes easier to read, I tried to avoid putting "GF" or "gluten free" in front of most condiments although I recognize that some of the brands may contain gluten while others are gluten free. The choice of brands will be up to the reader. I also tried to avoid brand names, but where I did call for one, always check that ingredient's label, because names and ingredients change from year to year and from country to country. For example, a pumpkin product that is gluten free in the United States may in Canada become pumpkin pie mix containing gluten, while the label is almost identical. In Canada, icing sugar may contain gluten, while in the United States our powdered or confectioner's sugar is blended with cornstarch. The actual ingredients in products can change even within the United States from east to west.

I realize that many of the pies and cakes and some of the casseroles are high in calories, but they are no more so than those same dishes made with gluten. Many newly diagnosed celiacs need the extra food energy in order to regain weight lost during illness before the diagnosis. Some, like myself, may be able to tolerate more calories for a long period before the ability of their gut to absorb seems to return to normal. Only in the last few years have I had to worry about weight gain. If you have that problem, do as I now do; serve smaller portions of desserts, and reserve the rich casseroles for special occasions or share them with friends.

An easy way to reduce calorie intake is to revise your recipes by reading magazines and newspapers and noting the changes in "light" recipes when placed beside the "old" recipe. Butter is replaced with canola oil; cream becomes milk or evaporated nonfat milk; the number of eggs is lowered; cream cheese is changed to low-fat cottage cheese; the amount of sugar is cut; and sometimes the quantity of another ingredient is lowered, thus making the serving portions smaller.

Whether you use the recipes as written or alter them to fit your dietary needs, I hope you will enjoy using *More* (recipes) *from the Gluten-free Gourmet* to expand the limited diet to include tasty gluten-free dishes that can be enjoyed by family and friends.

B. H.

ACKNOWLEDGMENTS

Writing a cookbook is a shared experience. This one would never have taken form without a lot of help from others. I owe deep thanks to the following:

Helen Hauschild, Elaine Monarch, and Rosie Wartecker for assisting in medical research.

Betty Wason, Rita Nicoll, and Susan Kidd, cooking teachers, for their valuable suggestions on foreign cooking.

The food editors of papers and magazines, especially the *Seattle Times*, the *Seattle Post-Intelligencer*, the *Sacramento Bee*, *Bon Appétit*, *Better Homes and Gardens*, *Best Recipes*, and *Sunset*, for ideas about the latest in food trends and healthy eating.

The McCormick/Shilling Spice Company and Crescent Foods, Inc., for supplying information and literature on spices, herbs, and condiments.

My testers, who not only tested the recipes but fed them to family and guests. Special thanks go to two friends: Donna Jo Doepkin, who insisted I start this book, created several recipes, and tested about one-fourth; and Mary Gunn, who furnished recipes, read every recipe, and tested most. I will be forever grateful to the other testers, some of whom I have never met except by letter or phone call, for taking twenty or more recipes: Alys Carrasco; Penny Coffin; Robert Conklin; Carol Dolan; Deborah Groesbeck; Elsie Janthey; Mary and Katelynn Kiefer; Katherine Losch; Loretta Malloy; Janis Petrich; Janet Rinehart; Pam Templeton; Debbie Turner; Margaret Voelker; Joe

Warren; and Eleanor Westling. A final heartfelt thanks to Gerald Koblenz for being my bread machine tester.

Elaine Hartsook, R.D., Ph.D., and the Canadian Celiac Association for suggestions and a careful medical review of this book.

My writing group, which is still waiting for my "Great American Novel."

Finally, to my wonderful editor, Beth Crossman, for her unwavering faith in this book.

FOREWORD

This foreword is written from my viewpoint as a pediatrician, nutritionist, and celiac. I and others have benefited from the identification and avoidance of the celiac's "poisons"—collectively called glutens.

Celiac sprue was first reported in the first or second century by Aretaeus, a Cappadocean. He noted that bread did nothing to stop the wasting away of the sufferers. Samuel Gee accurately detailed the disease in 1888, and prophetically suggested "if the patient can be cured at all, it must be by means of diet." In 1918, Still lectured that "one form of starch which seems particularly liable to aggravate symptoms is bread." In 1950, William Dicke, a Dutch pediatrician, reported that the symptoms of celiac disease (CD) "are elicited or aggravated by certain types of flours, especially wheat and rye flours." Treatment of children with a diet without wheat, rye, barley, and oats spread rapidly and replaced the popular ten-bananas-a-day diet, but it took years before the gluten-free diet was accepted for adults.

The most recent landmark in CD history was 1989, when Holmes and his coworkers reported the signficant reduction of gastrointestinal malignancies and lymphomas as the remarkable benefit of a gluten-free diet in patients they had observed over twenty years.

Gluten-sensitive enteropathy, or celiac disease, is activated by unidentified environmental and genetic factors at any stage of life from infancy to adulthood. CD is characterized by a primary small intestine mucosal injury associated with ingestion of specific protein fractions in wheat, barley, oats, and rye causing malabsorption of most nutrients. Today's research tends to target the cause to be an unusual, enhanced, complex immune response recognized primarily by jejunal mucosal injury of the small bowel in genetically susceptible individuals, primarily of northern European heritage.

The common clinical CD symptoms are a painful, often rumbling, gassy and bloated abdomen with the classic foamy, foul, pale floating stools, or an uncomfortable nagging constipation with excessively bulky stools, or years of a myriad of vague symptoms of undue fatigue, irritability, anemias—both iron and folic acid—bone pain, burning feet, muscle weakness, and depression or lassitude. Headaches may occur after ingestion of any of the celiac-toxic glutens.

For those celiacs whose disease takes the form of dermatitis herpetiformis (DH), symptoms are a distressing burning, itching, painful outcropping of lesions over the face, scalp, neck, elbows, knees, buttocks, and other specific sites. Seventy to 80 percent of DH individuals, who also have some gastrointestinal injury, will benefit from a gluten-free diet.

Celiac disease has an 8 to 20 percent prevalence—both suspected and unsuspected—at any one time in the sons, daughters, brothers, and sisters of the celiac disease patient. The incidence of the disease in the United States is estimated to be one in every 2,500, with considerably higher figures for Ireland, England, Scotland, and parts of Europe of one in every hundred to one in every 600.

The small bowel biopsy is the standard for diagnosis of the gluten-sensitive enteropathy of CD and DH. A duodenal biopsy may be obtained under direct vision using a fiber-optic endoscope by swallowing a biopsy capsule.

Forty or more alcohol-soluble protein fractions (more specifically called gliadins and prolamins in wheat, known as secalins in rye, hordeins in barley, and avenins in oats) are collectively referred to as "glutens." These protein fractions are found in the plant kingdom subclass of monocotyledonous plants (monocots), which are members of the grass family of *wheat, oats, barley, rye, and triticale* (manmade cross of wheat and rye), and their derivatives, such as malt, grain starches, hydrolyzed vegetable/plant proteins, textured vegetable proteins, grain vinegars, some soy sauces, some binders and fillers in vitamins or prescription medications, and some "natural" flavorings.

Rice and corn, other members of the grass family, appear to be harmless. Less common grasses (sorghum, millet, teff, ragi, and Job's tears) are closely related to corn but have not been adequately studied to determine their absolute safety for CD- or DH-susceptible patients.

A disease controlled by avoiding a particular offending food substance sounds like a snap to handle. But gluten products and by-products are sneakily ubiquitous in our food chain. Lobbying for complete ingredient lists in food labeling is an ever-persistent endeavor. Many individuals, both scientists and laypersons, as well as active celiac groups in the United States and Canada, deserve our gratitude for their fine work in this area.

A celiac must become an expert in label reading and must reread labels on every trip to the store. It is unfortunately true that companies change ingredients in a product, and an item that may have been safe can change. The fillers and binders in medications, vitamin preparations, and over-the-counter drugs can be a source of gluten toxicity. Ask your pharmacist to call the manufacturer to verify that your medication is a gluten-free product. This is especially important in this age of generic equivalents.

Not all gastrointestinal discomforts are gluten related. Some may be due to food allergies, such as strawberries, shellfish, spices, dairy proteins, nuts, citrus fruits, chocolate, or to a lack of enzymes as seen in lactose intolerance or intolerance to sorbitol (a nonmetabolizable sugar) found in many sugar-free items from toothpaste to chewing gum to apple juice. Bacterial overgrowth in the small intestine, a gastrointestinal malignancy, or a deficiency of pancreatic enzymes must also be considered and treated. You should also remember that the response of the small bowel to many foods can be altered by stresses associated with infections, surgery, cancer, drug therapy, pregnancy, secondary malabsorption from CD/DH, and emotional trauma.

If you are having a recurrent diet-related problem, try to ferret out the offending food by writing down everything you are eating for a week or two. Don't forget your medications, candy, and all snacks. Note the brand name, the number of times you eat the foods, and the symptoms you may be having.

You should know that CD patients are at a higher risk for contracting severe infectious diarrheas and the complications associated with them. Salmonella, Camphylobacter, and Giardia are but a few such diseases from poorly cooked or stored foods or from water. It is wise to avoid unpasteurized dairy products and fresh cheeses as well as raw or minimally cooked fish, fowl, pork, or beef. Raw honey is not advised, particularly for babies, older persons, and anyone prone to constipation, in order to avoid neurotoxicity and fatalities associated with botulism.

To be a wise, healthy traveler, use only bottled or boiled water or milk, eat well-cooked hot foods, and eat only fruits that you can peel yourself with a clean knife after washing the peel well.

Osteoporosis and dental problems for celiacs may be a result of years of poor intake and/or malabsorption of calcium, phosphorus, magnesium, and Vitamin D and K. Nutritional anemias may be due to poor absorption of iron, plus other minerals and vitamins.

There are other disorders thought to have an immunological basis that are more prevalent in CD patients *and* their relatives. Such disorders include thyroid disease, asthma, pulmonary diseases, rheumatoid arthritis, Sjogren's syndrome, serum IgA deficiency, glomerulonephritis, IgA nephropathy, insulin-dependent diabetes mellitus, vasculitis, systemic lupus erythematosis (SLE), ulcerative colitis, Crohn's disease, liver disorders, polymyositis, scleroderma, and sarcoidosis.

CD/DH patients have found that they are all too often "medical orphans" or are sent to a psychiatrist to be convinced that they are well, when they are actually being poisoned by their gluten-containing diet. The only solution is to be an informed patient, responsible for keeping your diet gluten free. Any local hospital or medical school library will be able to help you get copies of the articles listed here, and reference libraries are excellent resources.

The University of Southern California School of Medicine at Los Angeles has begun a Celiac Disease/Dermatitis Herpetiformis Center for diagnosis, consultation with private physicians and their patients, physician education, and research. It is this approach, and the establishment of other centers such as the Center for Digestive Diseases at the University of Iowa School of Medicine, that will improve the diagnosis and care for CD/DH patients. This should also educate our young doctors-in-training and specialists about CD/DH so that our relatives of the future will not be medical orphans.

More from the Gluten-free Gourmet is a superb guidebook to fine dining and the best of health for gluten-sensitive individuals. A grateful thank you to Bette Hagman for this splendid book. A gluten-free diet is for life!

—Betty Bernard, M.D.
Associate Professor of Pediatrics,
University of Southern California

SELECTED BIBLIOGRAPHY

Books

Cooke, W. T., Holmes G. K. T. *Coeliac Disease.* (New York: Churchill Livingston, 1984). This an excellent clinical resource for a comprehensive review of CD/DH.

Mearin, M. L., C. J. J. Mulder, editors. *Coeliac Disease: 40 Years Gluten-Free.* (Dordrecht / Boston / London: Kluwer Academic Press, 1991).

National Research Council. *Recommended Dietary Allowances.* Tenth edition (Washington, D.C.: National Academy Press, 1989). This can be ordered through any bookstore and is a good addition to your home library.

Medical Journal Articles

Holmes, G. K. T., P. Prior, M. R. Lane, D. Pope, and R. M. Allan. "Malignancy in Coeliac Disease—Effect of a Gluten-free Diet." *Gut* 30 (1989): 333–38.

Kelly, C. P., C. F. Feighery, R. B. Gallagher, and D. G. Weir. "Diagnosis and Treatment of Gluten-Sensitive Enteropathy." *Advances in Internal Medicine* 35 (1990): 341–64.

Pasternack, A., P. Collin, J. Mustonen, et al. "Glomerular IgA Deposits in Patients with Celiac Disease." *Clinical Nephrology* 34, no. 2 (1990): 56–60.

Patel, D. G., C. M. E. Krough, and W. G. Thompson. "Gluten in Pills: A Hazard for Patients with Celiac Disease." *Canadian Medical Association Journal* 133 (1985): 114–15.

Trier, J. S. "Medical Progress: Celiac Sprue." *New England Journal of Medicine* 325 (1991): 1709–20.

Walker-Smith, J. A., S. Guandalini, J. Schmitz, D. H. Schmerling, and J. K. Visakorpi. "Revised Criteria for Diagnosis of Coeliac Disease." *Archives of Disease in Childhood* 65 (1990): 909–11.

LIVING WELL WITHOUT WHEAT

Almost twenty years ago I was diagnosed with nontropical sprue (one of the older names for celiac disease), and I still feel it's one of the best things that's happened to me.

Most people would never agree that being told they harbored an uncurable disease could be a good thing; but I was elated to find the real reason for the diverse and often debilitating ailments I'd suffered over many years. I was relieved to learn that I had a disease with a name and was not just imagining the symptoms, as the psychiatrists to whom I'd been referred had been telling me; I was even happier to hear I didn't have cancer, the symptoms of which the disease can imitate—weight loss, change in bowel habits, pain, malnutrition, mental fatigue.

I now realize this feeling of relief is common to almost every celiac when *finally* diagnosed.

When I was given two smudged diet sheets and told that that was all I needed for remission, I could have kissed the doctor. He promised no more bloating, diarrhea, and pain. After the many years of on-and-off suffering, all I had to do was stick to a diet—no wheat, oats, barley, or rye. I could do that, couldn't I?

I soon discovered the diet was not to be an easy one. "No gluten" sounds simple, but the "thou shalt nots"—not eat bread, not have pasta, not taste a cake (even for a birthday)—had thereby consigned me to a lifetime of plainly cooked meats, vegetables, and fruits.

Naturally, I didn't stick to the diet. It seemed too simple; I cheated and ate some bread and—after recovering from the consequences—

swore I would never do that again. But I would manage to have bread, somehow. Cakes, as well. That was pure cussedness on my part. I had never been a cake eater, but now that I couldn't have it, I even craved a piece. The only trouble was, at that time, I was a dedicated noncook.

Twenty years ago, I couldn't find any company baking breads for celiacs or those who had to avoid wheat. I discovered some all-diet breads that contained no sugar, no eggs, no milk, no gluten, and very little flavor. But the loaf looked like bread. For several years I ate this plus some dry-as-dust muffins I concocted from potato starch and rice flour. The cookbooks of the time contained no satisfactory recipes for baking with rice flour. This I discovered to my dismay as I turned out inedible mess after mess, consigned, after one taste, to my omnivorous garbage disposal.

I considered myself a writer, kitchen duty a necessary evil. I'd always picked my bread from the grocery shelf and stirred up any party cake from a mix. As for pies, even my poodle—who would eat anything as long as it was "people food"—carried my crusts to the backyard and buried them.

With the diagnosis, I had to make some changes. I joined celiac organizations and exchanged baking-disaster stories with others and listened for any hints on living with this disease. I learned, to my surprise, that if I cheated, even without any symptoms of poisoning, I could still be damaging my gut. Thus, I was forced to cook if I wanted to enjoy eating, and in so doing, got hooked on experimenting. I haven't stopped.

Gluten Free but Still Having Symptoms?

That was my problem. A few months into my diet, I knew I was eating gluten free but still had distress at times. My doctor suggested I stop eating dairy products for a while and test myself later by putting them back into my diet by starting with Cheddar cheese (because of its low-lactose content). Wise doctor!

If you still don't feel well after maintaining a strict gluten-free diet, there can be a logical answer. Perhaps you, too, have another food sensitivity.

One of the most common (at least immediately after diagnosis) is lactose intolerance. The symptoms of bloating and diarrhea after eating milk products may not cause damage to the villi (the lining of the intestines), but they can be most uncomfortable. Lactose intolerance for some can be transient and pass after the villi heal; in others it can persist. For either kind of intolerance, there are products such as Lactaid and Dairy Ease to help overcome the distress. There are also many good substitutes for milk in markets and health food stores. When I specify nondairy liquids in my recipes, they can be soy based, corn based, nut based, or rice based; all work in the recipe.

Certain celiacs have reported to me that they are also intolerant of or allergic to corn and corn products, soy and soy products, and eggs. These basic foods do not contain gluten but, since they are used widely in the celiac's diet, you might be blaming gluten for distress symptoms when they are actually caused by one of these foods.

There are many other foods (chocolate, shellfish, citrus, apples, peanuts, MSG, and so on) that can cause symptoms resembling gluten poisoning. If you think you have an allergy to these or others, the best way to discover the culprit for yourself is to recall all the foods you ate just before the attack and eliminate them one at a time.

A much more unusual problem is one easily corrected. Some celiacs, especially when first diagnosed, reported distress from too much fiber. In their effort to avoid gluten in bread, cakes, cookies, and pastas, they had eaten more nuts, seeds, rice bran, vegetables, and raw fruit than the damaged intestines could comfortably handle. By including gluten-free breads and pasta and changing to white rice for a short period, the symptoms disappeared and they could gradually increase their fiber without distress.

What Does the Future Hold for the Celiac?

The future looks good. With the many wonderful gluten-free flours readily available today and the growing number of companies dedicated to filling our needs, we celiacs can all live very well without wheat (and oats, barley, and rye).

The only requirement is that we stick to our gluten-free diet for life. What other incurable disease calls for such an easy prescription for living well?

The good health we achieve will also help us fight off other ailments and help us live as long as anyone whose health has not been ravaged by the disease.

In the United States we have several celiac associations with local support groups working to dispense information and advice, so the celiac need never feel isolated by a "rare" disease, as described in old medical texts. CD was once considered only a childhood ailment that could be outgrown. Now medical research has discovered that, although symptoms might disappear during adolescence, the disease is still present, and the villi will show damage if gluten is reintroduced into the diet.

Last year the concerted effort of dedicated members of celiac organizations across the country finally brought our little-known disease to the attention of Congress, and a section of an appropriations bill directs the National Institute of Health to allocate funds for research on celiac disease.

Research is confirming some suspected facts about this auto-immune disease. Through checking our own genetic backgrounds, we might find others in our families who have suffered similar symptoms and thus help a doctor reach a diagnosis faster, and perhaps keep others from hearing, "It's all in your imagination."

Although biopsy is still the only definitive diagnostic tool, research has pinpointed certain factors appearing in blood tests that can alert doctors to the possibility of the disease.

The only treatment remains a gluten-free diet, but I still feel fortunate in being diagnosed. Just as the doctor promised, I've had almost twenty years of what I call my second life and a far richer one than my first. The diet is not restrictive anymore. We can have exciting and tasty baked goods, whether we bake them ourselves or buy them from one of the growing numbers of suppliers (see page 343). We can make pastas and casseroles, once thought forbidden, and, thanks to the incredible new bread machines, we can make dozens of freshly baked breads with little more effort than the punch of a button.

Eating Away from Home

All of this is true when eating at home; all of this changes when we step out the door.

Eating in a restaurant is frustrating but not impossible. I've learned to ask the server or chef what is in that soup, that salad, that good-looking meat dish. At first, I felt a bit paranoid questioning this way; however, I not only saved myself from a painful gluten reaction, but discovered that servers are often interested in learning what *gluten free* means.

Dining in the homes of friends takes more finesse. I often call the hostess ahead of time, suggesting I bring a dish to share. If she declines with her meal all planned, I snack before I go so I can enjoy the company even if I do have to pass on any dish that might contain gluten.

It's easy to plan foods and cook gluten free when traveling in an RV or camping in a park. Another easy way of traveling is on cruise ships. I take my own bread and turn it over to the maître d' to keep in the freezer and bring out at meals, and I keep gluten-free cookies in my stateroom for that sweet snack. For bus tours, I carry my own crackers, pretzels, granola, some bread, many cookies—all made from recipes in this book. I extend these with purchased rice crackers, dried fruit, GF jerky, hard cheese, and carefully selected candies.

Some airlines offer gluten-free meals, but I still carry some bread, cheese, and a few cookies in my carryon in case the order for a special meal never reached the airline kitchen or in case I miss my connection—both of which have happened to me.

The Hospital Stay

One of the hardest visits to plan for is the short one in a hospital. There the celiac or wheat-allergic patient is at the mercy of often-overworked kitchen help who don't always know what is in the dishes on your tray. If you are going to the hospital, here are some suggestions:

If your hospital stay is planned, talk to the head dietician before you enter and ask that some gluten-free breads and cookies (in sealed packages) be ordered from a supplier (and the packages not be opened until you break the seal).

Avoid ordering foods that look like gluten-containing foods. For example, Cream of Wheat and Cream of Rice look alike to a sick person flat in a hospital bed (and to the harried help in the hospital kitchen). Ask for one of the gluten-free dry cereal, and demand it come to you with the seal on the box unbroken.

If you have no chance to plan ahead for your stay, my strongest advice is to ask before you eat, to question anything you don't recognize. Don't eat mixed dishes such as casseroles. Stick to Jell-O, baked potatoes, fruit, plain vegetables and meat, milk (if you are not lactose intolerant), coffee, tea, and juices. It's not a great diet; but getting poisoned in the hospital is not what you came for. Remember, you'll even have to check your medications since many have a gluten or lactose base (see page 12).

For the most recent and complete medical information about celiac disease or to find a local support group, contact one of the following organizations:

American Celiac Society/Dietary Support Coalition, 59 Crystal Avenue, West Orange, NJ 07052-3570; phone (973) 325-8837.
Canadian Celiac Association, 190 Britannia Road East, Unit 11, Mississauga, Ontario L4Z 1W6, Canada; phone (905) 507-6208 or (800) 363-7296.
Celiac Disease Foundation, 13251 Ventura Blvd., Suite 1, Studio City, CA 91604-1838; phone (818) 990-2354; fax (818) 990-2397.
Celiac Sprue Association/United States of America (CSA/USA), PO Box 31700, Omaha, NE 68131-0700; phone (402) 558-0600.
Gluten Intolerance Group of North America (GIG), 15110 10th Avenue SW, Suite A, Seattle, WA 98166; phone (206) 246-6652.
Internet: http://celiac@maelstrom.stjohns.edu/.
http://rdz.acor.org/lists/celiac/index.html

REFERENCES

Hartsook, Elaine. "Celiac Sprue in the '90s. Progress and Hope." Keynote address at the annual meeting of the Gluten Intolerance Group of North America, May 1990.

———. "How to Have a Successful Hospital Stay." Address at the Celiac Experience I, May 1991.

Holmes, G. K. T., P. Prior, M. R. Lane, D. Pope, and R. N. Allan. "Malignancy in Coeliac Disease—Effect of a Gluten-free Diet." *Gut* 30 (1989): 333–38.

Poetkau, Margaret. "Gluten Free but Still Sick." Address at Annual Conference Canadian Celiac Association, May 1991.

Seely, Stephen, David L. Freed, Gerald A. Silverstone, and Vicky Rippere. *Diet-related Diseases: the Modern Epidemic.* London, England, and Westport, Conn.: Croom Helm, AVI, 1985.

Sullivan, Stephen. "How Much Gluten Is Too Much?" Keynote address at Annual Canadian Celiac Association, May 1990.

Trier, J. S. "Medical Progress, Celiac Sprue." *New England Journal of Medicine* 325, no. 24 (Dec. 1991): 1709.

HIDDEN GLUTENS

Most celiacs quickly learn to recognize gluten in the wheat-flour base of breads, crackers, baked goods, and pastas. They learn to put on magnifying glasses in order to read labels on condiments and products like corn bread (made with some wheat flour), hot dogs with grain fillers, cereals that include barley malt. All of those product labels list a grain containing toxic glutens.

What celiacs new to the diet often don't realize is that toxic grains can hide under different names and labels. Some are not labeled at all and often are not discovered until a celiac reports a reaction to a researcher. Others have found there is enough gluten in their work environments to cause toxic reactions—some to the point of having to change employment.

In this chapter I am repeating my list of hidden glutens from *The Gluten-free Gourmet* and adding newly uncovered sources for gluten in foods and the environment. Some of these are, admittedly, very low in toxic content and might not cause trouble except to those who are exceptionally intolerant; but anyone on a gluten-free diet should be aware of the possibility of getting poisoned from sources they never expected.

Those who must avoid wheat or gluten should also be aware that although *some* condiments such as mayonnaise, pasta sauces, and soy sauces are gluten free, many contain a form of hidden gluten. We must read labels from one purchase to the next, since manufacturing companies often change formulas, and sometimes the light or cholesterol-free version will contain gluten while the regular style of the same brand is gluten free.

For a complete list of foods that are safe for a gluten-free diet and foods to avoid, please see the Gluten-free Diet on page 339.

HIDDEN GLUTENS
(Listed in *The Gluten-free Gourmet*)

Candy

The ingredients in candy must be listed on the label, but currently companies are not required to list any product that may dust the block on which the candy is rolled for shaping. Some do use wheat flour.

Caramel Color

Caramel color can be made from dextrose (corn), invert sugar, lactose, molasses, or sucrose (beet or cane). These are gluten free. Caramel color made in the United States and Canada is made from these sources. Imported items containing caramel color can be made from malt syrup or starch hydrolysates, which can include wheat. If in doubt of the caramel color used in an imported food product, contact the company for information.

Coffee (Instant or Powdered)

There should be no gluten in plain instant coffee manufactured in the United States or Canada, but some flavored coffees may contain the forbidden grains. I discovered on a European trip that powdered coffees sometimes caused distress symptoms. Freeze-dried coffees seem less apt to cause problems.

Decaffeinated Coffee

Although the process of decaffeinating should not include the use of gluten, some celiac sufferers have felt distress upon drinking decaffeinated coffee. Rather than gluten, the culprit could be the chemicals used in the process. Water-processed decaffeinated coffee does not seem to provoke symptoms. The warning about flavored coffee applies to flavored decaffeinated coffee also.

Dextrin

Can be made from corn, potato, tapioca, rice, or wheat; it might be wise to avoid dextrin unless it is labeled as corn dextrin, tapioca dextrin, and so on. To confuse one even more, malto-dextrin is made from cornstarch. It is often found in hot dogs, spaghetti sauce, and so on.

Envelopes and Stamps

Some pastes and glues can contain wheat products. It will not take many licks on envelope flaps that contain a wheat paste before one starts feeling distress. To be safe, buy a sponge-topped bottle made for sealing envelopes, fill it with water, and let it do the licking for you. (The U.S. post office now issues some self-adhesive stamps requiring no wetting.)

Flavorings and Extracts

Some of these are made with grain alcohol from a forbidden grain. You can easily substitute ethyl vanillin or dried orange or lemon peel for these flavors. There are also several lines of gluten-free flavorings. Look for them in health food stores or order by mail (see page 343).

French Fries

Plain french-fried potatoes made at home or ones cooked in separate oil in a restaurant should be safe, but beware of any place that fries the potatoes in hot oil also used for breaded products such as fish or chicken. Some of the bread particles may transfer to the potatoes. Beware, too, of spicy fries or other seasoned potatoes. They can contain bread or wheat crumbs. Note also that some frozen potato products list wheat on the labels. This is used to preserve the fresh look of the frozen product. Some restaurants use this trick to keep them white before cooking. Ask!

Hash Browns, Eggs, and Hamburger Patties

These could be gluten free, but, when ordering in a restaurant, be sure they are cooked on a clean griddle, not on one that has been used for frying pancakes and french toast or browning hamburger buns. Again, the gluten can transfer to your food. Be sure the hamburger is pure meat that doesn't include any questionable additives and that your hash browns don't contain wheat flour. Again, ask!

Hydrolyzed Vegetable Protein (HVP) and Hydrolyzed Plant Protein (HPP)

These can be derived from soy, corn, rice, peanuts, or casein from milk. They could also come from wheat. If you wish to use a product containing HVP or HPP, check with the manufacturer to find the source of the protein. HVPs and HPPs are found in many canned mixed foods—soups, sausages, and hot dogs, for example.

Imitation Seafood

Although imitation seafood is started with a gluten-free base of sirimi, a starch binder—cornstarch, potato starch, wheat starch, or wheat flour—is added to create the shape and look of lobster, crab or scallops. Be sure to read the label before purchasing imitation seafood. There are many GF imitation seafoods on the market. Call your nearest seafood dealer and ask him to name by brand those that are sold in your area. They are different from east to west and in Canada.

Even more dangerous to those intolerant of wheat is the tendency in restaurants to mix imitation with real seafood in salads and other dishes. Always ask if any imitation seafood has been used before ordering a crab, lobster, or scallop dish in a restaurant or deli.

Modified Food Starch

If listed on the food label in the United States, this starch could be corn, tapioca, or potato starch—all safe. But it frequently is wheat starch, the most common form of thickener. Check with the manufacturer to ascertain what form of starch is used. If it says *starch*, in the United States, this is *cornstarch*. Canadian labels usually list "modified starch" with its derivative such as corn, tapioca, potato, or wheat.

Prescriptions (and Over-the-Counter Drugs)

Most tablets, lozenges, and capsules use a filler, which can be cornstarch, wheat starch, or lactose. The wise celiac will check all prescriptions with the doctor or pharmacist. If the filler of the medication ordered is a substance containing gluten, a substitute brand might prove to be gluten free. Sometimes a different medication can be prescribed.

A large number of prescriptions use a lactose base and, since many celiacs suffer from lactose intolerance, these, too, can cause bloating, diarrhea, gas, or other celiac-like distress symptoms. In spite of the seeming toxicity and uncomfortable reaction, this distress doesn't damage the villi as would gluten. If a substitute cannot be found, some patients can avert reactions by taking Lactaid or Dairy Ease tablets with their lactose-based drugs.

Rice Syrup

This flavoring can contain barley malt and might cause trouble for a celiac. If in doubt about the source of the rice syrup, write to the company for exact information.

Tea

Tea is on the celiac's safe drink list, but some patients have complained that instant teas have induced discomfort. Again, the problem could be something else in the powdered product. Remember to read the labels on herb and flavored teas for additives that may contain gluten.

Triticale

This grain found in some cereals and some flour mixtures is a cross of wheat and rye and contains toxic gluten.

MORE HIDDEN GLUTENS

Other grains that celiacs should avoid are *bulgar* (wheat that has been boiled, dried, and cracked), *spelt* (sometimes called German wheat, it is closely related to other wheats), *semolina* (the wheat from which much pasta is made), *durum flour* (another name for a hard wheat flour), and *couscous* (a wheat-grain semolina). For rice couscous products that are acceptable on our diet, see page 343 for suppliers.

Vegetable Sprays

Vegetable sprays are an excellent way of cutting fat out of frying, but not all such sprays on the market are gluten free. Always read the label to make sure the one you purchase is safe. One, especially made for baking, contains a large percentage of wheat.

Wheat Starch

A warning: Some products list wheat starch rather than wheat flour in the ingredient list. Avoid this as you would wheat flour. Although the starch part of wheat is not the most toxic factor, and some older cookbooks for celiacs contain recipes using wheat starch, it is not allowed by the medical experts in either the United States or Canada because of the impossibility of eliminating all the gluten when making wheat starch. (In England, wheat starch is allowed on the gluten-free diet.)

Gluten in the Workplace

Celiacs have become ill by breathing in and swallowing gluten while at work or doing a hobby that they never suspected was dangerous. For example:

A drywall construction man became ill sanding seams. He discovered the seaming paste contained wheat. A similar thing happened to a do-it-yourselfer who tried to finish her own walls.

A photographic worker continued to have toxic symptoms even on a GF diet until his doctor realized the films he sorted at work were separated with wheat flour.

A baker retired because of the amount of gluten present in the air at his workplace. A celiac who did a lot of baking to cater her friends' parties discovered that frequent baking with wheat flours caused her distress even though she did not eat any of the baked products.

FOR FURTHER CONSIDERATION

Distilled Vinegar

Safe for celiacs are cider, wine, or rice vinegars. Distilled vinegar is being researched, but although it is now allowed in Canada, it has not been removed from our forbidden list in the United States.

Veined Cheeses

Roquefort cheese was originally made by rolling bits of French bread into the cheese before putting it into the caves in Roquefort, France, for curing. Today some veined cheeses *may* use a cultured blue mold. The Dairy Council of Washington stated that the cheese companies would not share their formulas, but they admitted that although the molds are now cultured, they could be of bread origin. Whether these veined cheeses (blue cheese, Stilton, Gorgonzola, Roquefort) could contain enough gluten to be restricted on a celiac diet is still being researched.

DON'T CONTAIN GLUTEN, BUT SOUND LIKE IT

Buckwheat

Of the rhubarb family, not the grass family, buckwheat should be safe in products like kasha (pure roasted buckwheat kernels), but because it is used with other flours in baking, one should probably question any buckwheat flour. In every supermarket I checked, the so-called buckwheat flour was a blend of buckwheat and wheat. In health food stores, the label did not list ingredients, nor did it claim to be pure buckwheat flour.

Maltol

This is a synthetic flavoring substance. In spite of its name, it does not contain malt or gluten.

Monosodium Glutamate (MSG)

In the United States and Canada, MSG is produced from sugar beet molasses, so, for the celiac, there should be no concern about gluten poisoning when eating foods containing MSG (unless you are allergic to MSG and suffer distress from it).

Glutinous Rice (Sticky Rice)

The term *glutinous* means "gummy" and does not refer to any gluten content.

REFERENCES

Campbell, J. A. "Dialogue on Diet." *Celiac News*, Canadian Celiac Association, Ontario, Canada, Fall 1990.

———. "Diet Therapy of Celiac Disease and Dermatitis Herpetiformis." *World Rev. Nutr. Diet* 51 (1987): 189–233.

Ciclitira, Paul J. "A Vision for Future Research into Celiac Disease." Address at Annual Conference Canadian Celiac Association, Edmonton, Alberta, Canada, May 1991.

Cole, S. G. and M. F. Kagnoff. "Gluten-free Diet and Nutrition." *Annual Review of Nutrition* 5 (1985): 241–66.

Eekhof-Stork, Nancy. *The Great International Cheese Board*, pp. 30, 56. New York: Paddington Press, 1979.

Hartsook, Elaine. From lectures at the Celiac Experience, May 1991.

Kasarda, Donald D. "Toxic Proteins and Peptides in Celiac Disease: Relations to Cereal Genetics." In *Food, Nutrition, and Evolution: Food as an Environmental Factor in the Genesis of Human Variability*, edited by D. Walcher and N. Kretchmer, pp. 201–214. New York: Masson Publishing, 1981.

Layton, T. A. *The Cheese Handbook*, pp. 98, 115. New York: Dover Publications, 1973.

Liston, John. "From Seed to Shining Sea." Address on sirimi at Institute for Food Science, University of Washington (Seattle), November 1988.

Tyus, Frances J. "Additives . . . Knowing Can Make Your Diet More Flexible." Paper delivered at National CSA/USA convention, October 1988.

Winter, Ruth. *A Consumer's Dictionary of Food Additives*. Rev. ed. New York: Crown Publishers, 1984.

COOKING WITH GLUTEN-FREE FLOURS AND OTHER SUBSTITUTES

If you've turned out hockey pucks when baking muffins, crumbs in place of cookies, or lead instead of bread, you are well aware how "quirky" our gluten-free flours can be. Before the advent of xanthan gum, we used many eggs to stick the flours together, and we waited for the medical experts to come up with a pill to counteract our intolerance to gluten. That's still a dream, but we do have xanthan gum.

The protein (gluten) to which we are intolerant is also the stretch factor in the flours, so we have to add a substitute, which can be additional eggs, cottage or ricotta cheese, extra leavening, and xanthan gum (or guar gum) to make the baked product taste, look, smell and feel like "real." Cooking with gluten-free flours can seem tricky until one understands their limitations.

Rice flour is the basic flour for our diet, but I seldom bake with it alone. A better product results when rice flour is combined with other flours—potato starch, tapioca, or soy. A flour mixture and the addition of xanthan gum can make the food so tasty that no one will ever guess it's a diet product.

For my test baking and recipe converting, I start with a combination I keep on hand, GF flour mix (see page 22 for formula). Then I increase the eggs and leavening and add xanthan gum in a ratio of a little less than 1 teaspoon to a cup of flour in breads, 1/2 teaspoon to a cup of flour in cakes or muffins, and none in most cookies. Sometimes that is all that's needed. Other changes might be exchanging mayonnaise for oil or shortening for butter. But if the results aren't as good as I wish, I then deviate from the GF flour mix to achieve the desired texture. A higher ratio of tapioca flour makes a baked product more springy; potato starch flour, drier and tastier; soy, more moist and flavorful.

To satisfy your longing for sweets and breads, start with simple recipes if you are a noncook and haven't used these flours before. It won't be long before you turn out baked products that your non-dieting friends will envy. They'll never remember if you weren't much of a cook before. I know, for I was once in your shoes.

Because the flours do not exchange in equal quantity with wheat flour, it is best to understand what each flour is. And, because so many celiacs have other intolerances and allergies and must alter the formulas even more, I have listed some of the substitutes available for our dietary needs.

White Rice Flour

A white flour milled from polished white rice, this is the basic flour in my baking for it has a bland flavor that doesn't distort the taste of the baked product and combines well with other flours (to prevent the grainy texture of an all-rice cake or bread). White rice flour keeps well, so it can be bought in quantity. Order it through a supplier (see page 343) or buy it in unopened boxes (to avoid contamination) from bakeries, where it is used to dust baking pans. It is also available in many oriental markets.

White rice flour comes in several textures. Regular and fine can be ordered from suppliers, while the very finest is sold in oriental markets. All the recipes in this book were tested in my kitchen with fine rice flour of a medium grind from Ener-G-Foods. If using regular grind, you may have to add slightly more liquid; less liquid is needed for oriental flour.

Brown Rice Flour

A flour milled from unpolished rice, this contains the bran, and is higher in nutrient value than white rice flour. It is great for some breads, muffins, and cookies where the bran (or nutty) taste is desired, but, because there are oils in the bran, it has a much shorter shelf life and tends to become stronger tasting as it ages. Purchase fresh flour and store it in the freezer for a longer life.

Rice Bran

As the name implies, this is the bran obtained from polishing brown rice. It has a high content of minerals, vitamin B, vitamin E, protein, and fiber. I often add it to cookies, muffins, and some breads. This, too, has a short shelf life because of the oils it contains, so it is best to buy it as needed. Don't store it for long except in the freezer.

Sweet Rice Flour

This flour, made from a glutinous rice, often called sticky rice, is an excellent thickening agent. It is especially good for sauces that are to be refrigerated or frozen since it inhibits separation of the liquids. I have found this in many grocery stores in small boxes labeled as Mochiko Sweet Rice Flour, but it can be ordered from several of the suppliers listed on pages 343 to 347. It can also be found in some oriental markets. (Do not confuse it with plain white rice flour in the market.)

Rice Polish

A soft, fluffy, cream-colored flour made from the hulls of brown rice. Like rice bran, it has a high concentration of minerals and B vitamins. And, like rice bran, it has a short shelf life.

Potato Starch Flour

A very fine white flour with a bland taste, excellent for baking when combined with other flours, and a good thickening agent for cream soups. Use only about half the amount to replace wheat flour, and mix it with water before adding it to a soup. Potato starch flour keeps well and can be bought in quantity.

Potato Flour

Do not confuse this with potato starch flour. This is a heavy flour with a definite potato taste; I use very little of it. When called for in a recipe, potato flour can often be replaced with Potato Buds or mashed potatoes.

Tapioca Flour

Sometimes called tapioca starch, cassava flour, or cassava starch, this very light, white, velvety flour obtained from the cassava root imparts a bit of chew to baked goods and is excellent used in small quantities with other flours for most baking. I have also used it in almost equal parts in recipes where chew is desirable, such as French bread. This keeps well and can be bought in quantity.

Soy Flour

A yellow flour with high protein and fat content, this has a nutty flavor and is most successful when used in combination with other flours in baked products that contain fruit, nuts, or chocolate. With its distinctive taste, it is also excellent in waffles. Purchase soy flour in small quantities since it, too, has a short shelf life. Because there seem to be more celiacs sensitive to soy flour than to the white rice, potato starch, and tapioca flours, I don't use it in my GF flour mix. This can sometimes be purchased in a low-fat version.

Cornstarch

A refined starch obtained from corn, it makes a clear thickening for puddings, fruit sauces, and oriental dishes. Cornstarch is also used in combination with other flours in baking.

Corn Flour

A flour milled from corn (maize), this can be blended with cornmeal when making corn breads and corn muffins.

Cornmeal

This ground corn may be obtained in yellow or white meal. Combine this with other flours for baking or use it alone in Mexican dishes.

Arrowroot Flour

Especially desirable for those allergic to corn, this white flour obtained from the root of a West Indian plant can be exchanged measure for measure for cornstarch.

Nut Flours

Chestnut, almond, and other nut flours can be used in small quantities to replace a small portion of other flours in order to enhance the taste of homemade pasta, puddings, and cookies. Because they are expensive and often difficult to find, I did not use them in any recipes in this book. If you have the opportunity to experiment, they are great additions to the diet, for they are high in proteins.

Bean Flours

Garbanzo or other bean flours may be combined with rice flours for baking. They can also be added in small quantities to meat loaf, hamburger patties, and meatballs. I did not put in any recipes for these flours in this book, but they are high in food value and a great addition to the diet. Look for these in health food and East Indian stores.

GF Flour Mix

This is the basic mix I use in many recipes. The formula is two parts white rice flour, two-thirds part potato starch flour, and one-third part tapioca flour. I mix this in large quantities and keep it on hand for baking.

Example 1	Example 2
6 cups white rice flour	12 cups white rice flour
2 cups potato starch flour	4 cups potato starch flour
1 cup tapioca flour	2 cups tapioca flour

If you prefer not to blend your own, this flour can be ordered in boxes and bulk from one of the suppliers listed on pages 343 to 347. Ask for GF Gourmet Flour Mix or Bette Hagman's GF Gourmet Flour Mix.

PRINCIPLES OF SUBSTITUTION

For general baking, use the following formula. For each cup of wheat flour called for in a recipe, substitute *one* of the following:

> 1 cup of my GF flour mix, suggested above
> $7/8$ cup rice flour (brown or white)
> $5/8$ cup potato starch flour
> 1 cup soy flour plus $1/4$ cup potato starch flour
> $1/2$ cup soy flour plus $1/2$ cup potato starch flour
> 1 cup corn flour
> 1 scant cup fine cornmeal

Xanthan Gum

A powder milled from the dried cell coat of a microorganism called *Xanthomonas campestris* grown under laboratory conditions, it works as a substitute for the gluten in yeast breads and other baked goods using our gluten-free flours. It is available in some health food stores and by mail order from suppliers listed on pages 343 to 347.

Guar Gum

A powder derived from the seed of the plant *Cyamopsis tetragonolobus*. This can be purchased in health food stores or ordered from suppliers listed on pages 343 to 347. Because this has a high fiber content and is sometimes used as a laxative, one should be aware that when used in baking it can cause distress to people whose digestive systems are sensitive.

SUBSTITUTIONS FOR OTHER INTOLERANCES AND ALLERGIES

If you are lactose intolerant, in baking bread, substitute one of the powders found in health food stores: Lacto-Free or Tofu White (both contain soy) or NutQuik (made from almonds). Another choice could be a powdered baby formula from a supermarket or drugstore: Isomil, ProSobee, Nursoy (all soy based) or Pregestimil (corn based). For both drinking and cooking, there are several soy liquids in the dairy section of your local supermarket. You may also find a pure rice liquid called Rice Dream at many health food stores. This can be used directly from the box in place of milk.

If you must avoid all parts of the egg, use Egg Replacer (free of egg, dairy, corn, soy, gluten), mixing with water as suggested on the package. As in all our baking, you may have to increase the amount to get the desired texture of cake or muffins. I worked out one recipe for bread using Egg Replacer (see Egg Replacer Bread, page 56).

For those allergic only to egg yolks or cutting down on cholesterol, use Eggbeaters (contains egg whites) according to package directions or use egg whites in place of whole eggs. Use two egg whites for one egg or three for two eggs. Replacement works best when only one or two eggs are called for in a recipe.

Many of the recipes may be further altered to fit other dietetic needs. *The diabetic* can replace sugar with sugar substitutes. In baking, the results are better if the substitute sugar is used in heavier, moister cakes and breads (Pacific Rim Cake, page 100, or Fruit and Fiber Muffins, page 83). *Those who cannot tolerate soy* can replace soy flour in a recipe with rice flour. Since soy creates a more moist batter, you may need slightly more liquid if you exchange it.

For those who must lower their sodium intake, herbs and spices, light salt, or salt substitute can replace some or all of the salt. But *always read the labels on your mixed or substitute seasonings*; some contain anticaking agents in the form of wheat flour or germ. Some of the cheeses can be exchanged for varieties lower in sodium. You can buy "light" chicken and beef broths and stocks or make your own salt-free versions using only herbs for seasoning, and keep them in the freezer to use later.

Anyone who needs more fiber could substitute brown rice flour for the white, add rice bran in many of the recipes, and include more high-fiber vegetables in the casseroles and soups.

If you prefer not to use wine, substitute a sparkling cider or grape juice. In some recipes where the wine is used to tenderize meat, try using a tablespoon or so of red wine vinegar. One tester used Diet 7UP as a tasty alternative.

The preceding may be confusing to someone just starting the diet, but the flours and alternatives for dairy products soon become as familiar as the various mixes previously pulled off the grocery shelves.

The cooking may consume a bit more time, but the results are worth it, especially when the whole family can eat (and enjoy) the same meal from soup through dessert.

THE INCREDIBLE
BREAD MACHINE

Two years ago I staggered into the kitchen and plunked my new electric bread baker on the kitchen counter.

My husband looked up and said, "I thought you didn't like making bread."

"I don't. This monster is going to do it for me."

I had no idea I'd soon be calling it "a little jewel" and touting it as "the handiest appliance in the kitchen." I was still overwhelmed by the electronic system and the promises in the direction manual— if I ever learned to push those magic buttons.

I wasn't ready to become an owner of this machine, but I'd been shamed into the purchase. I'd heard about electric bread bakers but hadn't investigated much. The week before, at a meeting of local celiacs where one bread machine was on display, a member leaned over to me and said, "Your True Yeast Bread works great in my machine, but it always runs over. Why?"

Another wanted to know if any of the other bread recipes worked. She hadn't tried them yet. The final blow was when they all wanted to know which machine I used.

I had to confess I didn't own a bread baker—yet. They couldn't have been more surprised if I'd admitted I still scrubbed clothes on a washboard.

To save face, the next day I went out to do some serious looking. I might not have had replies at the time, but I was sure I could find them for those who'd asked . . . and had left phone numbers for me to call with answers.

If you've been baking bread the old-fashioned way, as I had, and dreaded those endless hours of measuring, mixing, beating, rising, punching down, and the pouring into bread pans, doing another rising session (all the while keeping an even, warm temperature in the kitchen), and then the hour of baking, an electronic bread baker seems too good to be true. Advertising claimed all one had to do was toss the ingredients into a square, round, or loaf-shaped pan and push a button. Approximately four and one-half hours later, out comes a loaf of bread. For once, those advertising geniuses have not exaggerated. In fact, I thought the claims most sedate. For me, the auto-baker has proved to be one of the biggest timesavers in the house, and I still haven't pushed all the buttons.

Once you decide to invest in a bread machine, the next question to face is this: Do you have to have one that makes a loaf shaped exactly like the bakery loaf you are familiar with, or can you accept a square or round loaf? I would have taken Z-shaped bread to get out of baking twice a week—especially when I discovered that in my new climate-controlled condo, bread often came out a disaster. Chilly air-conditioning fighting the sun through the windows left the dough rising and falling like the tide outside and the bread as soggy as if it had been splashed by the waves.

The bread machine eliminates disasters by perfectly controlling the climate within the tiny metal box, but when we use gluten-free flours, it isn't quite as easy as the publicity claims. (So what is?) I find it is better to preblend the dry ingredients (except the sugar and yeast) and to premix the liquid ones separately outside the container. You will find these suggestions incorporated into all my bread recipes.

The real question is what machine works best with our difficult gluten-free flours. I worked with a fellow celiac, and we have come up with some answers that are based on the machines that turn out the 1 1/2-pound loaf using approximately 3 cups of flour. This is the most common machine and the one for which the recipes in this book are planned, but don't be surprised if your bread loaf is the right size but weighs considerably more. The one-pound machine also works, but all the recipes have to be cut down by one third.

1. All machines can turn out excellent bread. The ones that have the strongest stir power seem to work best with our batterlike dough. If the paddle (kneading blade) is strong and the sides have added ridges and/or inserts (kneading rods) to help blend the dough, the machine will turn out a fine loaf of bread. Before you purchase a machine, check to be sure that the paddle at the bottom is the same thickness for the full vertical length. The machines with paddles that are part wand and resemble a hook might require prebeating outside the baking pan to completely blend the dough, or the batter may need to be stirred while the machine is running. We discovered that the dough in the more loaf-shaped (oblong) container doesn't always get as well stirred in the corners as in the upright square or circular pan. See the diagrams on page 28.

2. It is desirable for the machine to have a strong fan for the cool-down cycle. (If it doesn't, you will have to remove the bread immediately after baking; it becomes soggy if left in the pan.)

3. Where will the machine stand in your kitchen? Will the controls be convenient and the vents free of obstruction? Since the machines have different shapes and placement of control buttons and vents, you'll be able to find one to fit your kitchen space. (Even as I write this, I see there are more models being offered.)

4. Look at the lining of the baking pan. Is the Teflon or inside coating of a quality good enough to ensure a nonstick surface for a long time? Will the whole unit be easy to clean? In some machines the pan and paddle and all the parts that touch the bread are removable for easy cleaning. This is especially important if you intend to use the machine for gluten-free and wheat breads interchangeably. In some, a part of the paddle (or rotor it fits over) cannot be removed to wash, making it more difficult to clean thoroughly. This is no real problem if you plan to use it *only* for gluten-free bread. Also check the element and the inside of the machine (I think of it as the oven part). Will a simple wipe of a wet sponge or paper towel remove the baking dust and any spillover?

5. Price. There are machines that fit the above qualifications in every price range, but some more expensive models may have extra features that are worth investigating—and other features that are completely unnecessary.

6. Extra features. The machine, to be most automatic, should have a cool-down cycle. This means you don't have to be home when the cycle ends, giving you even more freedom. It also prevents burned hands, for there is very little room to maneuver a hot pan of bread

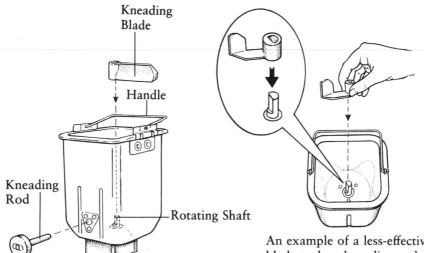

Kneading Blade

Handle

Kneading Rod

Rotating Shaft

This is an effective mixer for our heavy doughs. It has a good blade as well as a kneading rod.

An example of a less-effective blade and no kneading rod. This dough may need some hand stirring.

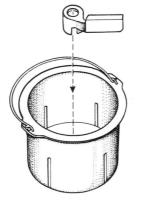

This model has a good blade but no kneading rod. The ridges in the pan aid in mixing dough.

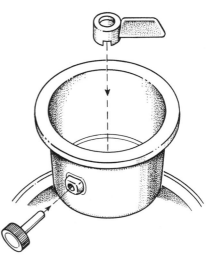

This is an example of a good blade with kneading rod. There is no handle on the pan.

Baking Pans and Parts

inside the machine. If the machine has a cycle at the beginning to heat the water or liquid, you will never have to wonder if your liquid is the right temperature (all ingredients are put in at room temperature). If the machine does not have this feature, my bread specialist suggests you never go wrong using warm (100°F to 110°F) for liquids.

Some automatic bread bakers have only two heats—light and dark. Others also have medium. Some call the levels by different names, such as sweet bread cycle (light) and white bread cycle (dark). After a little experience, the cook will become familiar with the cycles and learn to make his or her own judgment about what setting to use.

At least one machine can be programmed to different-length cycles—a great boon for those who need to have shorter rising times (in higher elevations, for example) and also good for experimenting with recipes.

My tester and I discovered no value in having a yeast dispenser, which doesn't work well with our flours. If you own such a unit, simply ignore this feature and place the yeast on the bottom of the pan before putting in the flour mix.

The time-delay feature of some bread machines is almost worthless for us since most of our gluten-free breads require eggs, and they should not stand for hours before baking.

Other advertising blurbs claim you can cook rice—or bake cakes, or make jam—in your bread makers. Don't let these come-ons tempt you. They do not make the best use of the machine.

Once I learned to push the buttons on my own bread maker, I started looking for the answers to my questions. Although every machine manufacturer provides a manual that answers some questions, there are still quirky things that happen with our flours.

Bread rises over or to top of pan and then falls. The reason could be too much yeast or water (or both). For automatic bread baking, I decrease the amounts of yeast and water.

You may use a different rice flour from Ener-G-Foods' fine white rice flour, which I used in testing all the recipes. Some flour sold as oriental rice flour is extra fine and needs less liquid. Try cutting down the amount of liquid 1 tablespoon each time you make a loaf until the desired result is achieved.

Using jumbo or extra-large eggs might cause the dough to be too thin. All my recipes were tested with large eggs. If you don't have this size, break them into a cup and use 2/3 cup eggs to equal 3 eggs.

Bread is very dry. Again, your flour can be to blame. Perhaps you have a coarser grind and need to add a little liquid, 1 tablespoon at a time, or you may have used more milk powder than the recipe calls for.

Center comes out doughy. Again, the problem can be too much liquid. Other possibilities are your machine was programmed to bake at too light a setting or for too short a cycle, or the circulation of air around the machine has affected the oven, or the bread dough didn't mix thoroughly before baking. If you have one of the machines with a large glass-domed top, try making an aluminum foil "hat" (shiny side facing in) to cover the top and enhance its insulation for better baking.

Dough doesn't mix thoroughly. Do you have one of the machines that doesn't have a strong paddle? Maybe you will have to assist the paddle by mixing with a rubber spatula in the first few minutes.

Another problem could be that the paddle is stuck. To avoid this, after every cleansing, rub a little vegetable oil in the hole where the paddle is placed over the rotor. If you haven't used the machine for a while, check that the paddle moves easily before placing ingredients in the pan.

Loaf doesn't round up like the picture in the manual shows. Don't be surprised at that. Mine doesn't either. My best-textured gluten-free loaf will be flat across the top. When I do achieve a rounded top, the texture tends to be dry and not springy.

Some bread recipes turn out a smaller loaf than others. If the texture is good, don't worry about the size. Some of the recipes, especially those using water or juice instead of milk or milk substitutes, do not contain as much protein, so don't rise as high.

Bread without eggs? I found we can make great-tasting bread using Egg Replacer, such as Egg Replacer Bread on page 56.

One of my testers has found an important breakthrough that will help you make a perfect loaf: one teaspoon unflavored gelatin dissolved in the liquids will greatly improve the texture of any bread made in a bread machine.

Probably the most important point is that my bread machine turns out delicious bread for myself, the family, and guests and I always bake gluten free. In fact, my husband prefers my breads to any he can purchase in the bakery or supermarket, and he never has regretted my dragging "that monster" into the house.

NOTE: I created nine specialty breads on pages 60 to 68 and the three sourdough breads on pages 70 to 72 especially for these marvelous new machines. Try them and see how they change your life.

BREADS

YEAST BREADS

Butter-Basted White Bread
Butter-Basted Brown and
White Bread
Tender Buttermilk Bread
Rapid-Rise French Bread
Russian Black Bread
Pumpernickel Bread
Sweet Swedish Mock Rye
Bread
Swiss Granola Bread
Russian Kulich
Apricot-Almond Bread
(Czechoslovakian)
Challah (Jewish Egg Bread)
Egg Replacer Bread
Rice Dream Bread (Lactose
Free, Soy Free, Corn Free)
Carrot-Bran Bread*
Apple-Spice Bread*

Orange-Pumpkin Bread*
Hawaiian Medley*
Mock Oatmeal Bread*
Boston Brown Bread*
Pink Onion Bread*
Popcorn Bread*
Buckwheat Bread*

SOURDOUGH BREADS

Simply Super Sourdough*
Italian Herb Sourdough*
Sandra's Mock Rye
Sourdough*

SHAPED YEAST BREADS AND ROLLS

Arab Pocket Bread (Pita
Bread)

*These great bread recipes were created specifically for baking with a bread machine but can also be made by conventional methods.

Crumpets (Lactose and
    Soy Free)
    Australian Toaster
        Buns
Ginger-Orange Rolls

SELF-RISING BREADS

Caraway Soda Bread
African Squash Bread
    Cream-Filled Squash
        Gems
Cranberry-Nut Bread
English Tea Scones (with
    Devonshire Cream)
    (with French Cream)

Grated Apple Loaf
Almond-Cheese Bread
    Almond-Cheese Muffins
Fruit and Fiber Muffins
Kiwi Muffins
Swedish Hardtack
Flaky Breakfast Rusks
Mock Graham Crackers

BREAKFAST BREADS

Drop Scones (Scotch
    Pancakes)
Raised Doughnuts
    Baked Doughnuts
Fruited Breakfast Torte

Although those great-smelling breads on your regular grocery shelf are still forbidden, gluten-free bread for celiacs has improved considerably since I was diagnosed twenty years ago. There are tasty breads to be ordered from suppliers and found in health food stores. Since the development by the nutrition department of the University of Washington (Seattle) of a recipe using xanthan gum, we can bake our own delicious yeast breads. With the increasingly popularity of the new automatic bread baking machines we can make them with almost no effort. (See "The Incredible Bread Machine," page 25.)

If you're still stuck on rice cakes as your only bread, browse this chapter. There are breads here, both yeast and self-rising, that rival any on your bakery shelf for flavor. I've adapted recipes to our flours for many national breads—from the Arabian pita bread and a wonderfully rich black Russian bread to a new quick-rising French bread. When I took a warm loaf of this to a new celiac, she broke off the top sticking out of the wrapper, popped it into her mouth, and exclaimed, "Why, it tastes just like real!"

Of course it does. Baking bread and having it come out tasting good can be very satisfying, but there are still some formulas for exchanging flours and increasing proteins that have to be learned, and even a few tricks I've discovered to have success with our often quirky flours.

Follow the mixing directions carefully (even if they sound weird).

Use fresh yeast. Yeast is dated on packages or jars. Don't try to save money using old yeast.

Use regular yeast, not quick rising unless the recipe calls for it. I prefer fresh yeast cakes for their flavor and easy digestibility, but, since they are often hard to find and difficult to keep fresh, I have worked out all the recipes in this book using 1 tablespoon dry yeast granules in place of the 1 cake fresh yeast. One packet of dry yeast is considered to be 1 tablespoon.

The water for softening the yeast must be only lukewarm. Too hot will kill the yeast; too cold, the yeast will not work. Test with a thermometer (105°F to 115°F) or put a drop on the inside of your wrist, as one tests milk for a baby's bottle. The water should contain some sugar. *If using a bread machine, follow the directions accompanying your machine for water temperature.*

A heavy-duty mixer (such as a KitchenAid) helps mix our bread. The dough is softer and stickier than gluten-bread dough and cannot be kneaded by hand; but, since it is a thick dough, it can burn out motors on light mixers if used often. Always used the heavy-mixer paddle rather than the dough hook on the machine unless otherwise instructed.

Rice flours may be milled to different textures (see page 18). Each texture will take a slightly different amount of water when used in baking bread. The following recipes were tested with Ener-G-Foods' fine rice flour, which is between regular and extra fine of oriental rice flours. You may have to add 1 to 2 tablespoons more liquid if you use regular flour, and omit 1 to 2 tablespoons if using oriental rice flour.

Baking time and temperature for all breads was based upon conditions at sea level. Bread should be tipped gently from pan to cool immediately upon removing from oven. To test for doneness tap gently at the bottom of the loaf. It should sound hollow. If the sides cave in slightly or the bread does not seem done, return pan to oven for 5 or more minutes. If using a bread machine, and the loaf seems underbaked, place it on a baking sheet and place it in a preheated 400° oven for about 5 minutes or until it tests done. (Next time try a higher setting on your machine.)

Xanthan gum is necessary for all the yeast recipes to help make the breads springy and chewy. It replaces, in part, the gluten that rice and potato flours lack. This is available in some health food stores and from the suppliers listed on pages 343 to 347.

Guar gum may be substituted for the xanthan gum in equal amounts, but guar gum, often sold as a laxative, may cause distress to some. Guar gum is available in health food stores.

Let the bread dough rise in a warm place. Putting the pan in an oven that has been heated to 200° and then turned off works well. Another trick is to set the mixing bowl in a pan or sink full of warm water.

Adding extra protein in the form of eggs, dry milk solids, or cottage cheese helps the yeast work. The formulas in this book have been perfected through much trial and error. If you must change ingredients, remember that you must have protein in some form. Soy powder substitutes for milk powders contain the required protein; so does NutQuik, the nut substitute. Ricotta cheese can often be substituted for cottage cheese.

A teaspoon of GF vinegar added to any yeast bread recipe helps the yeast work and develops flavor. Vinegar may be replaced by gluten-free dough enhancer, available in many health food stores and some kitchen supply stores. Dough enhancer is wonderful for making bread tender, more flavorful, and long lasting. However, it may contain ingredients to which some people are allergic, hence I list vinegar as the first choice. Use 1 tablespoon for the dark breads and 1 teaspoon for the light ones. Always add this to the liquids, not to dry ingredients.

Milk powder, unless otherwise specified, is noninstant dry milk powder. Unlike the instant granules readily available on the grocery shelf, this is found in health food stores and in some large markets. Nonfat, noninstant milk powder is excellent, but the regular gives more milk flavor (and more fat) to bread. If you cannot find any noninstant milk powder, you may substitute the regular instant dry milk, but this changes the formula.

In some recipes I've listed Egg Replacer as optional. I find this makes the texture of all baked goods better, so I use 1 to 1¹/₂ teaspoons of this in all my baking, for breads, cakes, and waffles, etc. This may be purchased in health food stores or ordered from Ener-G-Foods (see the list of suppliers on pages 343 to 347).

Baking the bread in small pans (2¹/₂" × 5") or muffin tins will often turn out a product with better texture.

The eggs used in all the recipes in this section are large size unless otherwise specified. Jumbo, extra-large, medium, or small eggs will change the formula. Each large egg is slightly less than $1/4$ cup, so if you have eggs of a different size, break the eggs into a measuring cup and use $2/3$ cup to equal 3 eggs.

A combination of gluten-free flours is the final secret of the good taste in many of the recipes. A formula that works successfully for much of my baking is my GF flour mix. You can purchase it from some suppliers (see pages 343 to 347) or mix it yourself.

The formula is: 2 parts white rice flour
$2/3$ part potato starch flour
$1/3$ part tapioca flour

YEAST BREADS

BUTTER-BASTED WHITE BREAD

Tastes like a wheat bread, looks like a wheat bread, smells like a wheat bread. This variation of my original True Yeast Bread is not as sweet but is buttery tasting and much more tender. You may substitute 3 cups of GF flour mix (see above) for the three separate flours listed. Bread-machine directions follow hand-mixing directions.

2 cups white rice flour
$1/2$ cup potato starch flour
$1/2$ cup tapioca flour
$2^1/2$ teaspoons xanthan gum
$2/3$ cup dry milk powder
  (or $1/2$ cup nondairy
  substitute; see Note)
$1^1/2$ teaspoons salt
$1^1/2$ teaspoons Egg
  Replacer (optional)
3 tablespoons sugar, divided

$2/3$ cup lukewarm water
$1^1/2$ tablespoons dry yeast
  granules
4 tablespoons ($1/2$ stick)
  butter or margarine,
  melted
1 additional cup warm water
1 teaspoon vinegar or
  1 teaspoon dough
  enhancer
3 eggs, room temperature

Combine the flours, xanthan gum, milk powder, salt, Egg Replacer (if used), and all but 2 teaspoons of the sugar in bowl of a heavy-duty mixer. Use your strongest beater, not the bread hook.

Dissolve the remaining sugar in the 2/3 cup of lukewarm water and mix in the yeast.

Combine the melted butter with the cup of water; add the vinegar or dough enhancer.

Turn mixer on low. Blend the dry ingredients and slowly add the butter-water mixture. Then add the eggs one at a time. This mixture should feel slightly warm.

Pour the yeast mixture into the bowl and beat at the highest speed for 2 minutes. Place the mixing bowl in a warm spot, cover with plastic wrap and a towel, and let the dough rise in a warm place for approximately 1 hour, or until doubled.

Return the dough to the mixer and beat on high speed for 3 minutes (see Note). Spoon dough into three 2¹/₂" × 5" greased loaf pans or 1 large pan. Fill 2/3 full. You may bake the remainder in muffin tins. Or make all rolls (approximately 18; see Note).

Let the dough rise until it is slightly above the top of the pan, 45 to 60 minutes. Preheat oven to 400°. Bake the large loaf for approximately 1 hour, small loaves slightly less, and rolls for about 25 minutes. Cover with foil after 10 minutes of baking. To test breads for doneness, tap gently with finger. Bread will have a slightly hollow sound. Remove from pan immediately to cool.

NOTES: The dough texture will seem more like cookie dough than bread dough, so don't be alarmed.

This bread has a finer texture when baked in small loaf pans and is delicious in rolls. You can easily double the recipe to turn out 2 large loaves plus 18 rolls or 3 small loaves plus 24 rolls. The bread freezes well. For convenience, slice before freezing.

For the lactose intolerant, see page 23 for nondairy substitutions.

BREAD MACHINE: Combine the flours, xanthan gum, milk powder, and salt. Measure the sugar. Beat the eggs.

Combine *all* the water, the butter, vinegar, and eggs. (If your machine manual recipes call for warm water, use that. If it has a preheating cycle, put in at room temperature.)

Cut the amount of yeast to 1 tablespoon.

Place the ingredients in the baking pan of the bread maker in the order suggested in your manual. (Some place yeast on bottom, flour mix next, then sugar and liquids; other suggest the reverse order.)

Use the white bread setting at medium crust (if you have this selection).

BUTTER-BASTED BROWN AND WHITE BREAD: Exchange 1 cup or both cups of the white rice flour for brown rice flour. The results are excellent.

TENDER BUTTERMILK BREAD: A tasty bread with a distinctive flavor, it seems to stay fresh longer than other breads. Some lactose-intolerant celiacs can use buttermilk, so this may be a boon for them if they are allergic to the soy in some of the baby formulas or the coconut oil in most of the nondairy substitutes.

Follow the recipe for Butter-Basted White Bread, but substitute 1/2 cup powdered buttermilk for the milk powder and omit the vinegar. Follow directions for hand mixing or making with the automated bread machine.

RAPID-RISE FRENCH BREAD

Crusty outside, soft and tender within, this quick and easy French bread formula uses rapid-rise yeast and requires only one rising. You can make it, from start to finish, in about one hour. Serve hot from the oven and watch everyone rave.

2 cups white rice flour	2 tablespoons rapid-rise
1 cup tapioca flour	yeast
3 teaspoons xanthan	2 tablespoons butter or
gum	margarine, melted
1 1/2 teaspoons salt	3 egg whites, beaten
2 teaspoons Egg Replacer	slightly
(optional)	1 teaspoon vinegar
2 tablespoons sugar	Melted butter, for brushing
1 1/2 cups lukewarm water	(optional)

In the bowl of a heavy-duty mixer, place flours, xanthan gum, salt, and Egg Replacer (if used). Blend with mixer on low.

Dissolve the sugar in the water and add the yeast. Wait until the mixture foams slightly, then blend into the dry ingredients. Add the butter, egg whites, and vinegar. Beat on high speed for 3 minutes.

To form loaves, spoon dough onto greased and cornmeal-dusted cookie sheets in two long French-loaf shapes or spoon into special French-bread pans. Slash diagonally every few inches. If desired, brush with melted butter.

Cover the dough and let rise in a warm place until doubled in bulk, 20 to 25 minutes. Preheat oven to 400°. Bake for 40 to 45 minutes. Remove from pan to cool. *Makes 2 loaves.*

RUSSIAN BLACK BREAD

A delicious bread wonderful with soups or stews, Russian Black Bread is great also with cheese or fish spreads on your appetizer table. The secret of the flavor comes from the chocolate and coffee added to the more usual seasonings.

2 cups GF flour mix
3/4 cup brown rice flour
1/2 cup rice bran or Brown Rice Cereal (uncooked)
2 teaspoons caraway seeds
1 teaspoon freeze-dried coffee crystals
1/2 teaspoon onion powder
2 1/2 teaspoons xanthan gum
1 1/2 teaspoons salt
1/2 cup dry milk powder or nondairy substitute
1 1/2 tablespoons cocoa powder
3 tablespoons sugar, divided

3/4 cup lukewarm water
1 1/2 tablespoons dry yeast granules
1 additional cup warm water (scant)
3 tablespoons vegetable oil
2 tablespoons molasses
1 teaspoon vinegar or 1 1/2 tablespoons dough enhancer
3 large eggs, room temperature
1/2 teaspoon cornstarch and 1/4 cup water, for brushing (optional)

In the bowl of a heavy-duty mixer, place the flours, rice bran, caraway seeds, coffee crystals, onion powder, xanthan gum, salt, dry milk powder, cocoa, and all but 2 teaspoons of the sugar. Blend on slow speed.

Dissolve the remaining two teaspoons of sugar in the 3/4 cup lukewarm water and add the yeast. Set aside to foam.

In the additional cup of water stir together the oil, molasses, and vinegar (or dough enhancer).

With mixer on low speed, blend the water-yeast liquid into the dry ingredients. Add the oil-water mixture and then break in the eggs, one at a time. Turn to high and beat for 2 minutes.

Cover the bowl and set in a warm place for 1 to 1 1/2 hours, or until dough is doubled in bulk. Return bowl to the mixer and beat another 2 minutes. Fill one 2¹/₂" × 5" greased tin ²/₃ full. Form the rest of the dough into a ball shape and place in a greased 8" casserole. Allow the dough to rise for 40 to 50 minutes, or until doubled in bulk. Preheat oven to 350°. Bake for 25 to 30 minutes for the small loaf tin, and 40 to 50 minutes for the casserole loaf.

Boil the cornstarch with ¹/₄ cup of water for about 30 seconds in a saucepan over high heat. While still hot, brush the loaves with the cornstarch mixture. Let cool on wire rack before slicing.

BREAD MACHINE: Combine the flours, rice bran, caraway seeds, coffee crystals, onion powder, xanthan gun, salt, milk powder, and cocoa. Set aside. Measure the sugar. Beat the eggs.

Combine *all* the water, the oil, molasses, vinegar, and beaten eggs (if your machine directions suggest warm, use warm water; if machine has preheating cycle, use room-temperature water).

Cut the amount of yeast to 1 tablespoon.

Place the ingredients in the baking pan of the bread maker in the order suggested in your manual. (Some place yeast, then flour, then sugar, and then liquids; other suggest the reverse order.)

Use the white bread setting at medium crust (if you have this selection).

PUMPERNICKEL BREAD

This absolutely wonderful, chewy bread tastes like that gluten-laced pumpernickel some of us remember. And it stays tender for days—if you can keep it from the rest of the family—so is great for lunch sandwiches. Bake it in small pans and slice thin for your appetizer tray with pâtés and spreads.

2 cups brown rice flour
1/3 cup tapioca flour
2/3 cup potato starch flour
2 1/2 teaspoons xanthan
  gum
3 teaspoons caraway seeds
1 1/2 teaspoons salt
1/2 cup dry milk powder or
  nondairy substitute
1 tablespoon cocoa powder
3 tablespoons sugar,
  divided

2/3 cup water, lukewarm
1 1/2 tablespoons dry yeast
  granules
7/8 cup (14 tablespoons)
  additional warm water
3 tablespoons molasses
1 teaspoon vinegar or
  1 tablespoon dough
  enhancer
2 tablespoons vegetable oil
3 eggs, beaten lightly

In the bowl of a heavy-duty mixer, combine flours, xanthan gum, caraway seeds, salt, milk powder, cocoa, and all but a couple of teaspoons of the sugar. Use your mixer's strongest beater, not the bread hook.

Dissolve the remaining sugar in the 2/3 cup lukewarm water and mix in the yeast. Set aside while you combine the additional water, molasses, vinegar, and oil.

Turn mixer to low speed and blend the dry ingredients. Slowly add the oil-water liquid. Blend. Add the eggs. The dough should feel slightly warm. Add yeast water and beat at highest speed for 2 minutes. Cover, mixer and all, with a towel and let the dough rise in a warm place for approximately 1 hour, or until doubled.

Beat again for 3 minutes. Spoon dough into three 2 1/2" × 5" greased and rice-floured loaf pans or 1 large pan plus several muffin tins. Fill all 2/3 full.

Let dough rise, covered, in pans until it is slightly above the top of the pans, 45 to 60 minutes. Preheat oven to 375°. Bake the large loaf for approximately 1 hour, small loaves slightly less, and muffins for about 25 minutes.

BREAD MACHINE: Combine the flours, xanthan gum, caraway seeds, salt, milk powder, and cocoa. Set aside. Measure the sugar. Beat the eggs.

Combine *all* the water, the molasses, vinegar, oil, and eggs. (If your machine directions suggest warm water, add warm water. Add at room temperature if your machine has a preheating cycle.)

Cut the amount of yeast to 1 tablespoon.

Place the ingredients in the baking pan of the bread maker in the order suggested in your manual. (Some add yeast, then flour, then sugar, and then liquids; other suggest the reverse order.)

Use the white bread setting at medium crust (if you have this selection).

SWEET SWEDISH MOCK
RYE BREAD

There are many variations of Swedish rye bread, but this one tastes so similar to the one served at my in-laws' family gatherings that they all thought I'd used wheat and rye flours. A great "company" bread and equally good for sandwiches with mild-tasting fillings that don't overpower the wonderful flavor of the bread, this bread makes up well by hand or in the bread machine.

2 cups brown rice flour
2/3 cup potato starch
   flour
1/3 cup tapioca flour
2 1/2 teaspoons xanthan
   gum
1/2 cup Isomil powdered
   baby formula (see
   Note)
1 1/2 teaspoons salt
2 teaspoons dried lemon
   peel
1 teaspoon cardamom
1/2 cup dark brown sugar,
   divided
2/3 cup lukewarm water

1 1/2 tablespoons dry yeast
   granules
4 tablespoons (1/2 stick)
   butter or margarine,
   melted
7/8 cup (14 tablespoons)
   additional warm water
1 teaspoon vinegar or
   1 tablespoon dough
   enhancer
2 tablespoons light
   molasses
1 teaspoon almond
   flavoring
3 eggs, room temperature

In the bowl of a heavy-duty mixer, combine flours, xanthan gum, Isomil, salt, lemon peel, cardamom, and all but a couple of teaspoons of the sugar. Use your mixer's strongest beater, not bread hook.

Dissolve the remaining sugar in the 2/3 cup lukewarm water and mix in the yeast. Set aside while you combine the butter, additional warm water, vinegar, molasses, and almond flavoring.

Turn mixer to low speed and blend the dry ingredients. Slowly add the butter-water liquid. Add the eggs. The dough should feel slightly warm. Add yeast water and beat at highest speed for 2 minutes. Cover, mixer and all, with a towel and let dough rise in a warm place for approximately 1 hour, until doubled.

Beat again for 3 minutes. Spoon dough into three 2½″ × 5″ greased and rice-floured loaf pans or 1 large pan plus several muffin tins. Fill all ⅔ full.

Let dough rise, covered, until it is slightly above tops of pans, 45 to 60 minutes. Preheat oven to 375°. Bake the large loaf for approximately 1 hour, small loaves slightly less, and rolls for about 25 minutes.

NOTE: If you don't use Isomil, substitute noninstant dried milk powder; also replace 1 tablespoon of the brown rice flour with 2 tablespoons soy flour. The soy adds to the flavor. If you are allergic to soy, the bread turns out successfully with the dry milk powder but has a slightly different flavor.

BREAD MACHINE: Combine the flours, xanthan gum, Isomil, salt, lemon peel, and cardamom. Set aside. Measure the sugar. Beat the eggs.

Combine *all* the water, the butter, vinegar, molasses, almond flavoring, and eggs. (If your machine directions suggest warm water, add warm water. Add at room temperature if it has a preheating cycle.)

Cut the amount of yeast to 1 tablespoon.

Place the ingredients in the baking pan of the bread maker in the order suggested in your manual. (Some place yeast, then flour, then sugar, and then liquids; others suggest the reverse order).

Use the white bread setting at medium crust (if you have this selection).

SWISS GRANOLA BREAD

A tender-textured, nutty bread. Wonderful for sandwiches. It tastes best with the combination of brown and white flours suggested, but if you don't have these, you may substitute 3 cups of GF flour mix and add ¹/₄ cup rice bran.

1 cup brown rice flour
1 cup white rice flour
¹/₂ cup potato starch flour
¹/₂ cup tapioca flour
1 cup granola (page 189), ground fine
2¹/₂ teaspoons xanthan gum
1¹/₂ teaspoons salt
²/₃ cup dry milk powder or ¹/₂ cup nondairy substitute
1¹/₂ teaspoons Egg Replacer (optional)

3 tablespoons sugar, divided
²/₃ cup lukewarm water
1¹/₂ tablespoons dry yeast granules
4 tablespoons (¹/₂ stick) butter or margarine, melted
1 additional cup water
1 teaspoon vinegar or 2 teaspoons dough enhancer
3 eggs, room temperature

In the bowl of a heavy-duty mixer, combine flours, granola, xanthan gum, salt, dry milk, Egg Replacer (if used), and all but 2 teaspoons of the sugar. Use your mixer's strongest beater, not a bread hook.

Dissolve the remaining sugar in the ²/₃ cup lukewarm water and mix in the yeast. Set aside while you combine the butter with the additional cup of water and the vinegar.

Turn mixer to low speed and blend the dry ingredients. Slowly add the butter-water mixture. Add the eggs. This mixture should feel slightly warm.

Pour the yeast water into the ingredients in the bowl and beat at highest speed for 2 minutes. Place the mixing bowl in a warm spot, cover with plastic wrap and a towel, and let the dough rise for approximately 1 hour, or until doubled.

Return the dough to the mixer and beat on high speed for 3 minutes. The dough will seem more like cookie dough than bread dough, but don't be alarmed. Spoon the dough into three 2¹/₂" × 5" greased, rice-floured loaf pans or 1 large pan plus a few muffin tins. Fill ²/₃ full.

Let the dough rise in pans until it is slightly above the tops of the pans, 45 to 60 minutes. Preheat the oven to 375°. Bake the large loaf for approximately 1 hour, small loaves slightly less, and muffins for about 25 minutes.

BREAD MACHINE: Combine the flours, granola, xanthan gum, salt, milk powder, and Egg Replacer (if used). Set aside. Measure the sugar. Beat the eggs.

Combine *all* the water, the butter, vinegar, and beaten eggs. (If your machine manual calls for warm water, add warm water. Add at room temperature if it has a preheating cycle.)

Cut the amount of yeast to 1 tablespoon.

Place the ingredients in the baking pan of the bread maker in the order suggested in your manual. (Some add yeast, then flour, then sugar, and then liquids; others suggest the reverse order.)

Use the white bread setting at medium crust (if you have this selection).

RUSSIAN KULICH

Sweet, moist, and fruit filled, this bread is a holiday treat in Slavic countries. The suggested orange glaze is optional. The nondairy substitutes give greater flavor, Isomil for soy, NutQuik for almond. If you don't have the flours listed, replace them with 3 cups of GF flour mix.

2 cups white rice flour
1/2 cup potato starch flour
1/2 cup tapioca flour
1 tablespoon xanthan gum
1/2 cup Isomil or NutQuik
    nondairy powder (finely
    ground in food
    processor)
1 1/2 teaspoons salt
1 teaspoon dried lemon
    peel
1/3 cup sugar, divided
2/3 cup lukewarm water

1 1/2 tablespoons dry yeast
    granules
4 tablespoons (1/2 stick)
    butter or margarine,
    melted
1 additional cup water
1 teaspoon vinegar or
    dough enhancer
1 teaspoon almond extract
3 eggs, room temperature
1/2 cup candied fruit mix
1/3 cup chopped toasted
    almonds (see Note)

ORANGE GLAZE

1 cup confectioner's sugar
1 tablespoon soft butter or margarine
2 to 3 tablespoons hot orange juice

In the bowl of a heavy-duty mixer, combine flours, xanthan gum, Isomil, salt, lemon peel, and all but 2 teaspoons of the sugar. Use your mixer's strongest beater, not the bread hook.

Dissolve the remaining sugar in the 2/3 cup lukewarm water and mix in the yeast. Set aside while you combine the butter with the additional cup of water, the vinegar, and almond extract.

Turn mixer to low speed and blend the dry ingredients. Slowly add the butter-water mixture. Add the eggs. The mixture should feel slightly warm.

Pour the yeast mixture into the ingredients in the bowl and beat at the highest speed for 2 minutes. The dough texture will seem more like cookie dough than bread dough, so don't be alarmed. Place the mixing bowl in a warm spot, cover with plastic wrap and a towel, and let the dough rise for approximately 1 hour, or until doubled.

Return the bowl to the mixer, add fruit mix and almonds, and beat on high speed for 3 minutes. Spoon the dough into three 2^1/$_2$" × 5" greased, rice-floured loaf pans or 1 large pan. Fill ^{2}/$_3$ full. Bake the remainder in prepared muffin tins.

Let the dough rise in pans until it is slightly above the tops of the pans, 45 to 60 minutes. Preheat oven to 375°. Bake the large loaf for approximately 1 hour, small loaves slightly less, and rolls for about 25 minutes. Cool before glazing (if desired).

To make the glaze (if used), mix together all ingredients until of a spreading consistency.

NOTE: To toast almonds, spread in a single layer in a shallow pan. Bake at 300° to 325° for about 10 minutes, stirring often. The nut-meats will change from ivory to tan and will continue to toast slightly after they are removed from the oven.

BREAD MACHINE: Combine the flours, xanthan gum, Isomil, salt, candied fruit mix, lemon peel, and almonds. Measure the sugar. Beat the eggs.

Combine *all* the water, the butter, vinegar, almond extract, and beaten eggs. (If your machine manual call for warm water, add warm water. Add at room temperature if your machine has a preheating cycle.)

Cut the amount of yeast to 1 tablespoon.

Place the ingredients in the baking pan of the bread maker in the order suggested in your manual. (Some add yeast, then flour, then sugar, and then liquids; others suggest the reverse order.)

Use the white bread setting at medium crust (if you have this selection).

APRICOT-ALMOND BREAD
(Czechoslovakian)

A sweet bread filled with dried fruit and doubly flavored with almond. Serve it for breakfast or brunch or pair it with a salad for a luncheon. Use firm dried apricots. The soft Turkish fruits tend to settle to the bottom rather than remain distributed throughout the loaf. You may substitute 3 cups of GF flour mix for the flours listed. For the bread machine method, you may use all apricot nectar instead of the water.

1 cup white rice flour
1 cup brown rice flour
1/2 cup tapioca flour
1/2 cup potato starch flour
3 teaspoons xanthan gum
1/2 cup NutQuik nondairy powder, ground fine (see Note)
1 1/2 teaspoons salt
1/3 cup brown sugar, divided
2/3 cup lukewarm water
1 1/2 tablespoons dry yeast granules

4 tablespoons (1/2 stick) butter or margarine, melted
1 cup apricot nectar
1 teaspoon almond flavoring
1 teaspoon vinegar
3 eggs, room temperature
1/2 cup chopped dried apricots
1/3 cup toasted almonds, chopped (see Note)

In the bowl of a heavy-duty mixer, combine the flours, xanthan gum, NutQuik, salt, and all but 2 teaspoons of sugar. Blend the dry ingredients on low speed.

Add the remaining sugar to the water and stir in the yeast. Let sit until it foams.

Combine the butter with the apricot nectar, add the almond flavoring and vinegar.

With mixer on low speed, blend in the water-yeast mixture. Add the butter-nectar mixture and break in the eggs, one at a time, beating after each addition. With mixer on high speed, beat for 2 minutes.

Cover the bowl and set in a warm place for 1 to 1¹/₂ hours, or until dough doubles in bulk.

Beat another 2 minutes. Stir in the apricots and almonds. Spoon dough into three 2¹/₂" × 5" greased and rice-floured loaf pans or 1 large pan. Fill ²/₃ full. If any dough remains, bake in greased muffin tins.

Let the dough rise until slightly above the tops of the pans, 45 to 60 minutes. Preheat oven to 375°. Bake for approximately 1 hour for a large loaf, about 45 minutes for small ones, about 25 minutes for rolls.

NOTE: NutQuik may be replaced with noninstant milk powder or a nondairy substitute, but with the loss of some of the almond flavor.

To toast almonds, spread in a single layer in a shallow pan. Bake at 300° to 325° for about 10 minutes, stirring often. The nutmeats will change from ivory to tan and will continue to toast slightly after they are removed from the oven.

BREAD MACHINE: Combine the flours, xanthan gum, NutQuik, salt, apricots, and almonds. Set aside. Measure the sugar. Beat the eggs.

Use one (12-ounce) can of apricot nectar plus enough water to make 1²/₃ cups. Combine this mixture with the eggs, vinegar, almond flavoring, and butter. (If your machine recipes suggest warm water, add warm water. Add at room temperature if it has a preheating cycle.)

Cut the amount of yeast to 1 tablespoon.

Place the ingredients in the baking pan of the bread maker in the order suggested in your manual. (Some place yeast, then flour, then sugar, and then liquids; other suggest the reverse order.)

Use the white bread setting at light crust (if you have this selection).

CHALLAH
(Jewish Egg Bread)

A delicious lactose-and-soy-free sweet bread topped with poppy seeds. This is often braided, but since our bread dough is too soft to handle well, I've given directions only for loaves.

2 cups white rice flour
1³/₄ cups tapioca flour
¹/₄ cup sugar, divided
3 teaspoons xanthan gum
1¹/₂ teaspoons salt
²/₃ cup lukewarm water
1¹/₂ cakes yeast or 1¹/₂ tablespoons dry yeast granules

4 tablespoons (¹/₂ stick) butter or margarine, melted
1 additional cup water
1 teaspoon vinegar
3 eggs plus 2 egg yolks
Poppy seeds (optional)

In the bowl of a heavy-duty mixer, combine the flours, sugar (reserving 2 teaspoons), xanthan gum, and salt. Use your mixer's strongest beater, not the bread hook.

Dissolve the remaining sugar in the ²/₃ cup lukewarm water and mix in the yeast.

Combine the butter with the additional cup of water and the vinegar.

With mixer on low speed, blend the dry ingredients. Slowly add the butter-water mixture. Blend in the eggs and yolks one at a time. The dough should feel slightly warm. Pour the yeast mixture into the ingredients in the bowl and beat at highest speed for 2 minutes. Place the mixing bowl in a warm spot, cover with plastic wrap and a towel, and let the dough rise approximately 1 hour, until doubled in bulk.

Return the dough to the mixer and beat on high for 3 minutes. Spoon the dough into three 2¹/₂" × 5" greased, rice-floured loaf pans or 1 large pan. Fill ²/₃ full. You may bake the remainder in greased muffin tins. Or make all rolls (approximately 18). Sprinkle tops with poppy seeds.

Let the dough rise until it is slightly above the tops of the pans, 45 to 60 minutes. Preheat oven to 400°. Bake the large loaf for approximately 1 hour, small loaves slightly less, and rolls for about 25 minutes.

BREAD MACHINE: Combine the flours, xanthan gum, and salt. Measure the sugar. Set aside. Beat the eggs slightly.

Combine the water to make 1²/₃ cups (if your machine suggests warm water, use that; if it has a preheating cycle, add water at room temperature). Add the butter, vinegar, and beaten eggs.

Cut the yeast to 1 tablespoon.

Place the ingredients in the baking pan of the bread maker in the order suggested in your manual. (Some place yeast, then flour, then sugar, and then liquids; others suggest the reverse order.) If you desire a poppy seed topping, sprinkle on after last rising in the machine before baking.

Use the white bread setting at medium crust (if you have this selection).

EGG REPLACER BREAD

A tasty bread for those allergic to or intolerant of eggs, this has a good texture and flavor. It can also be made soy and lactose free, if necessary, but the best bread is baked with noninstant milk powder. I have made this with 7UP as the liquid, so it can be egg, soy, corn, and lactose free and still taste good. You can easily double the recipe to turn out two large loaves plus eighteen rolls or three small loaves plus twenty-four rolls. The bread freezes well. For convenience, slice before freezing.

2^1/$_4$ cups rice flour (white or brown or mixed)

^{1}/$_2$ cup potato starch flour

^{1}/$_2$ cup tapioca flour

4 teaspoons xanthan gum

^{1}/$_2$ cup nonfat dry milk powder or nondairy substitute

1^1/$_2$ teaspoons salt

^{1}/$_4$ cup sugar, divided

^{1}/$_2$ cup lukewarm water

4 teaspoons dry yeast granules

4 tablespoons (^{1}/$_2$ stick) butter, margarine, or shortening, melted

1 additional cup lukewarm water

1 teaspoon vinegar

8 teaspoons Egg Replacer plus enough water to make ^{2}/$_3$ cup

^{1}/$_8$ teaspoon turmeric

In the bowl of a heavy-duty mixer, combine the flours, xanthan gum, milk powder, salt, and all but 2 teaspoons of the sugar. Use your mixer's strongest beater, not the bread hook.

Dissolve the remaining sugar in the ^{1}/$_2$ cup lukewarm water and mix in the yeast.

Combine the butter with the additional cup of water and the vinegar.

With mixer on low speed, blend the dry ingredients and slowly add the butter-water mixture.

Beat the Egg Replacer mixture with the turmeric and add to the batter. This should feel slightly warm.

Add the yeast mixture to the ingredients in the bowl and beat at highest speed for 2 minutes. The dough texture will seem more like cookie dough than bread dough, so don't be alarmed. Place the mixing bowl in a warm spot, cover with plastic wrap and a towel, and let the dough rise for approximately 1 hour, or until doubled.

Return the bowl to the mixer and beat on high for 3 minutes. Spoon the dough into three 2½" × 5" greased, rice-floured loaf pans or 1 large pan. Fill ⅔ full. You may bake the remainder in greased muffin tins. Or make all rolls (approximately 18). This bread has a finer texture when baked in small loaf pans and is delicious in rolls.

Let the dough rise until it is slightly above the tops of the pans, 45 to 60 minutes. Preheat oven to 400°. Bake the large loaf for approximately 1 hour, small loaves slightly less, and rolls for about 25 minutes.

VARIATION: Try adding ½ cup raisins or nuts, or 1 cup of finely chopped granola (see page 189), or ½ cup dried fruit (use some fruit juice in place of water). None of these additions will require more liquid.

BREAD MACHINE: Combine the flours, xanthan gum, milk powder, and salt. Measure the sugar. Beat turmeric with Egg Replacer and the water.

Combine the rest of the water (1½ cups), the butter, vinegar, and Egg Replacer mixture. (If your machine manual recipes call for warm water, then use that temperature water; if it has a preheating cycle, put in at room temperature.)

Reduce yeast to 1 tablespoon.

Place the ingredients in the baking pan of the bread maker in the order suggested in your manual. (Some place yeast, then flours, then sugar, and then liquids: others suggest the reverse order.)

Use the white bread setting at medium crust (if you have this selection).

RICE DREAM BREAD
(Lactose Free, Soy Free, Corn Free)

This tasty bread is for those who have multiple allergies in addition to gluten intolerance. Unlike the earlier breads created for all allergies and intolerances, this does contain sugar and salt, which give it great flavor. Rice Dream, the liquid suggested, can be purchased in many health food stores. The guar gum is preferable if you have a corn allergy.

2 cups rice flour (white or brown)
1/2 cup potato starch flour
1/2 cup tapioca flour
1/2 cup sweet rice flour
2 1/2 teaspoons guar (or xanthan) gum
1 1/2 teaspoons salt
2 teaspoons Egg Replacer (optional)
3 tablespoons sugar, divided

2/3 cup lukewarm water
1 1/2 tablespoons dry yeast granules
3 tablespoons canola or sunflower seed oil
1 cup Rice Dream (nondairy) liquid
1 teaspoon vinegar or 2 teaspoons dough enhancer (optional)
3 eggs, room temperature

In the bowl of a heavy-duty mixer, combine the flours, guar gum, salt, Egg Replacer (if used), and all but 2 teaspoons of the sugar. Use your mixer's strongest beater, not the bread hook.

Dissolve the remaining sugar in the 2/3 cup lukewarm water and mix in the yeast.

Combine the oil with the Rice Dream and vinegar or dough enhancer.

With mixer on low speed, blend the dry ingredients. Slowly add the oil–Rice Dream mixture. Blend. Beat in the eggs one at a time. The mixture should feel slightly warm.

Pour the yeast mixture into the bowl and beat at highest speed for 2 minutes. The dough texture will seem more like cookie dough than bread, so don't be alarmed. Place the mixing bowl in a warm spot, cover with plastic wrap and a towel, and let the dough rise for approximately 1 hour, or until doubled.

Return the bowl to the mixer and beat on high speed for 3 minutes. Spoon dough into three 2¹/₂″ × 5″ greased and rice-floured loaf pans or 1 large pan. Fill ²/₃ full. You may bake the remainder in muffin tins. Or you may prefer to make all rolls (approximately 18).

Let the dough rise until it is slightly above tops of pans, 45 to 60 minutes. Preheat oven to 400°. Bake the large loaf for approximately 1 hour, small loaves slightly less, and rolls for about 25 minutes. Cover with foil after 10 minutes of baking.

BREAD MACHINE: Combine the flours, guar gum, salt, and Egg Replacer (if used). Measure the sugar. Beat the eggs.

Use 1²/₃ cups Rice Dream, omitting the water, and combine with the oil, vinegar, and beaten eggs. (If your machine requires warm water, heat the Rice Dream to the recommended temperature; if it has a preheating cycle, add Rice Dream at room temperature.)

Cut the amount of yeast to 1 tablespoon.

Place the ingredients in the baking pan of the bread maker in the order suggested in your manual. (Some place yeast, then flour, then sugar, and then liquids; others suggest the reverse order.)

Use the white bread setting at medium crust (if you have this selection).

I created the following twelve exciting breads especially for the bread machine. Serve them at parties or luncheons. They're all so good that your gluten-eating friends will enjoy them, too. They can easily be made a day ahead; like all breads, they slice better when cold, and they're so moist they keep well.

CARROT-BRAN BREAD

Tasty, moist, and sweet without the use of sugar, this high-fiber bread could become one of your favorites. This has a heavy dough that you might wish to stir with a rubber spatula at the beginning of the mix cycle.

1 cup white rice flour
1 cup brown rice flour
$^1/_2$ cup potato starch flour
$^1/_2$ cup tapioca flour
$^1/_4$ cup rice bran
2$^1/_2$ teaspoons xanthan gum
$^1/_2$ cup noninstant dry milk powder or nondairy substitute
1$^1/_2$ teaspoons Egg Replacer (optional)
1$^1/_2$ teaspoons salt

1 teaspoon dried orange peel
1 cup finely grated carrots
3 eggs, beaten slightly
3 tablespoons honey
3 tablespoons oil
1 teaspoon vinegar or 4 teaspoons dough enhancer
1$^1/_2$ cups water
1 tablespoon dry yeast granules

Mix together the flours, bran, xanthan gum, milk powder, Egg Replacer (if used), salt, and orange peel. Blend in the grated carrots.

Mix together eggs, honey, oil, vinegar or dough enhancer, and water (warm or cool, as your bread maker's instructions suggest). Measure the yeast.

Place the ingredients in the baking pan in the order suggested in your manual. (Some start with the yeast and dry ingredients; others, with liquids, and then dry ingredients and yeast on top.) Use the machine setting at medium crust and adjust for the next loaf as necessary.

APPLE-SPICE BREAD

A delicious and different loaf for that next luncheon or dinner, this bread smells like apple pie while it's baking and hints of apple pie in its flavor. It is also wonderful toasted for breakfast or brunch. I suggest NutQuik or Isomil for the extra nutty taste, but you can substitute dry milk powder.

2 cups white rice flour
1/2 cup potato starch
   flour
1/2 cup tapioca flour
2 1/2 teaspoons xanthan
   gum
1 1/2 teaspoons apple pie
   spice
1 teaspoon dried lemon
   peel
1/2 cup NutQuik or Isomil
   nondairy substitute
1 1/2 teaspoons salt

1 1/2 teaspoons Egg
   Replacer (optional)
1 large apple, grated
1/4 cup sugar
1 tablespoon dry yeast
   granules
3 eggs, room temperature
1 1/2 cups water
3 tablespoons margarine or
   butter, melted
1 teaspoon vinegar or
   2 teaspoons dough
   enhancer

Combine flours, xanthan gum, spice, lemon peel, NutQuik, salt, and Egg Replacer (if used).

Peel, core, and grate the apple. Tumble it with the flour mix.

Measure the sugar and yeast.

Beat the eggs and combine with the water, margarine, and vinegar or dough enhancer. (If your machine manual calls for warm water, add warm water. Add at room temperature if your machine has a preheating cycle.)

Place the ingredients in the baking pan of your bread maker in the order suggested in your manual. (Some place yeast, then flour, then sugar, and then liquids; others suggest the reverse order.)

Use the white bread setting at medium crust and adjust for the next batch as necessary. This is a heavy dough, and you might want to stir with a rubber spatula just as the machine starts the mix cycle.

ORANGE-PUMPKIN BREAD

A dark, moist bread with a hint of pumpkin pie in smell and taste. The liquid is orange juice and water; the bran adds texture. For convenience I suggest using Junior squash for pumpkin.

1 cup white rice flour
1 cup brown rice flour
1/2 cup potato starch flour
1/2 cup tapioca flour
1/4 cup rice bran
2 1/2 teaspoons xanthan gum
1 1/2 teaspoons salt
3 teaspoons Egg Replacer (optional)
1 teaspoon pumpkin pie spice
Grated zest of 1 orange
1/2 cup chopped pecans (optional)

3 eggs, beaten
3 tablespoons butter or margarine, melted, or vegetable oil
1 teaspoon vinegar or 2 teaspoons dough enhancer
One 6-ounce jar Junior baby squash
Juice of 1 orange plus enough water to make 1 1/3 cups
4 tablespoons brown sugar
1 tablespoon dry yeast granules

Mix together the flours, bran, xanthan gum, salt, Egg Replacer (if used), spice, and orange zest. Stir in the pecans (if used).

Mix together the eggs, butter, vinegar, squash, and orange juice plus water (warm or cool, as your bread maker's manual suggests).

Measure the sugar and yeast.

Place the ingredients in the baking pan of your bread maker in the order suggested by your manual. (Some place yeast, then flour, then sugar, and then liquids; other suggest the reverse order.)

Use the light setting at medium crust and adjust for next loaf as necessary.

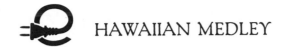 HAWAIIAN MEDLEY

A sweet fruit and nut bread with all the tastes of Hawaii. So good it can almost be dessert. Team it with fruit, fish, or chicken salads. If you don't have macaroon coconut, use dried coconut and chop finely in your food processor.

2 cups white rice flour
1/2 cup potato starch flour
1/2 cup tapioca flour
2 1/2 teaspoons xanthan gum
1 teaspoon dried lemon peel
1 1/2 teaspoons Egg Replacer (optional)
2 teaspoons salt
1/2 cup macadamia nuts, chopped
1/2 cup macaroon coconut

1/2 cup crushed pineapple, drained (reserve juice)
1 1/3 cups pineapple juice
4 tablespoons (1/2 stick) butter or margarine, melted
1 teaspoon vinegar or 1 1/2 teaspoons dough enhancer
3 eggs, slightly beaten
1/3 cup sugar
1 tablespoon yeast

Mix together the flours, xanthan gum, lemon peel, Egg Replacer (if used), and salt. Blend in the macadamia nuts, coconut, and pineapple.

Mix together juice (warm or cool, as your bread maker's manual suggests), butter, vinegar, and eggs.

Measure the sugar and yeast.

Place the ingredients in the baking pan of your bread maker in the order suggested by your manual. (Some place yeast, then flour, then sugar, and then liquids; others suggest the reverse order.) Use the machine setting at medium crust and adjust for the next loaf as necessary.

MOCK OATMEAL BREAD

This loaf has the taste, texture, and color of oatmeal bread with the addition of cinnamon and brown sugar. To crush the almonds, place in a plastic bag and crush with a rolling pin to the size of oatmeal.

1 cup white rice flour
1 cup brown rice flour
1/2 cup potato starch flour
1/2 cup tapioca flour
2 1/2 teaspoons xanthan
   gum
1/2 cup noninstant milk
   powder or nondairy
   substitute
1 1/2 teaspoons salt
1 1/2 teaspoons Egg
   Replacer (optional)
1 teaspoon cinnamon

1 cup sliced almonds,
   crushed
3 eggs, beaten slightly
1 2/3 cups water
4 tablespoons (1/2 stick)
   butter or margarine,
   melted
1 teaspoon vinegar or
   2 teaspoons dough
   enhancer
4 tablespoons brown sugar
1 tablespoon dry yeast
   granules

Mix together the flours, xanthan gum, milk powder, salt, Egg Replacer (if used), and cinnamon. Stir in the almonds.

Mix together the eggs, water (warm or cool as your bread maker's manual suggests), butter, and vinegar or dough enhancer.

Measure the sugar and yeast.

Place the ingredients in the baking pan of your bread maker in the order suggested by your manual. (Some place yeast, then flour, then sugar, and then liquids; others suggest the reverse order.)

Use the machine setting at medium crust and adjust for the next loaf as necessary.

BOSTON BROWN BREAD

A baked bread that tastes like our old steamed brown bread—moist, heavy, sweet, and delicious. Serve it with all the bean dishes or spread with butter and cream cheese for a dessertlike snack.

1 cup brown rice flour
1 cup white rice flour
1/2 cup potato starch flour
1/2 cup tapioca flour
3/4 cup popcorn flour or
   1/2 cup cornmeal
3 teaspoons xanthan gum
1/2 cup (scant) buttermilk
   powder
1 teaspoon baking soda
1 1/2 teaspoons Egg
   Replacer (optional)

1 1/2 teaspoons salt
2/3 cup raisins
3 eggs
1 teaspoon vinegar or
   1 tablespoon dough
   enhancer
2/3 cup molasses
4 tablespoons vegetable oil
1 1/3 cups water
2 tablespoons brown sugar
1 tablespoon yeast

Blend together the flours, xanthan gum, buttermilk powder, baking soda, Egg Replacer (if used), salt, and raisins.

Beat eggs slightly; add vinegar, molasses, oil, and water (warm or cool, as your bread maker's manual suggests). Blend thoroughly.

Measure the sugar and yeast.

Place the ingredients in the baking pan of the bread maker in the order suggested in your manual. (Some add yeast, then flour, then sugar, and then liquids; others suggest the reverse order.) Bake on regular bread setting on light or medium heat.

PINK ONION BREAD

A really different bread, great with cheese and meats such as corned beef or GF bologna. It's not really pink, but is peach colored. Pink Onion Bread uses 2 tablespoons of dry Onion Soup Mix (page 336) and 1 can of V-8 juice. This bread doesn't rise as high as other breads but is lactose, soy, and corn free.

1 cup brown rice flour
1 cup white rice flour
1/2 cup tapioca flour
1/2 cup potato starch flour
2 1/2 teaspoons xanthan gum
1 teaspoon salt
1 1/2 teaspoons Egg Replacer (optional)
2 tablespoons GF dry Onion Soup Mix (page 336)

3 eggs
1 teaspoon vinegar or 1 1/2 teaspoons dough enhancer
One 5 1/2-ounce can V-8 juice plus water to make 1 2/3 cups
3 tablespoons vegetable oil
3 tablespoons sugar
1 tablespoon dry yeast granules

Blend together the flours, xanthan gum, salt, Egg Replacer (if used), and soup mix.

Beat the eggs slightly; add the vinegar, V-8 juice and water (warm or cool, as your bread maker's manual suggests), and oil.

Measure the sugar and yeast.

Place the ingredients in the baking pan of the bread maker in the order suggested in your manual. Some place yeast, then flour, then sugar, and then liquids; others suggest the reverse order. Bake on light or medium.

POPCORN BREAD

A truly great, grainy-tasting bread, high in fiber. This uses a new flour created from popcorn (see suppliers listed on pages 343 to 347 for availability). Molasses and orange peel add extra flavor.

1 cup brown rice flour
1 cup white rice flour
3/4 cup popcorn flour
1/2 cup tapioca flour
1/2 cup potato starch flour
3 teaspoons xanthan gum
2/3 cup dry milk powder or
   1/2 cup nondairy
   substitute
1 teaspoon baking soda
1 1/2 teaspoons salt
2 teaspoons dried orange
   peel

1 1/2 teaspoons Egg
   Replacer (optional)
3 eggs
1 3/4 cups water
3 tablespoons vegetable oil
3 tablespoons molasses
1 teaspoon vinegar or
   2 teaspoons dough
   enhancer
2 tablespoons brown sugar
1 tablespoon dry yeast
   granules

Blend together the flours, xanthan gum, milk powder, soda, salt, orange peel, and Egg Replacer (if used).

Beat the eggs slightly; add the water (warm or cool, as your bread maker's manual suggests), oil, molasses, and vinegar. Blend.

Measure the sugar and yeast.

Place the ingredients in the baking pan in the order listed in your manual. (Some place yeast, then flour, the sugar, and then liquids; others suggest the reverse order.) Bake on light setting.

BUCKWHEAT BREAD

Fresh ground kasha (roasted buckwheat) flavors this delicious brown bread. By grinding your own kasha, you can be sure that there is no contamination in your "buckwheat" flour.

1 cup brown rice flour
1 cup white rice flour
1/2 cup tapioca flour
1/2 cup potato starch flour
1/2 cup kasha, ground
  slightly
2 1/2 teaspoons xanthan
  gum
1 1/2 teaspoons salt
1 1/2 teaspoons Egg
  Replacer (optional)

3 eggs
1 3/4 cups water
1 teaspoon vinegar or
  1 1/2 teaspoons dough
  enhancer
3 tablespoons vegetable oil
1 tablespoon molasses
3 tablespoons sugar
1 tablespoon dry yeast
  granules

Blend together the flours, kasha, xanthan gum, salt, and Egg Replacer (if used).

Beat the eggs slightly; add the water (warm or cool, as your bread maker's manual suggests), vinegar, oil, and molasses.

Measure the sugar and yeast.

Place the ingredients in the baking pan of the bread maker in the order suggested in your manual. (Some place yeast, then flour, then sugar, and then liquids; others suggest the reverse order.) Bake on regular bread setting on light or medium heat.

SOURDOUGH BREADS

Fresh yeast was not always available on the farm when I was young, so Mother kept a crock of "riser" going for her breads. I had absolutely no interest in baking then and so never realized this was a starter for what is now known as sourdough bread.

Today we can make fresh starter with purchased yeast any time we wish to make sourdough bread, but after tasting the following three breads, you might wish to imitate the farm wives (as I do now) and keep a crock of starter in the refrigerator all the time.

STARTER

> **Pinch sugar**
> **1 cup lukewarm water**
> **1 cake fresh yeast or 1 tablespoon yeast granules**
> **1¹/₂ cups white rice flour**

In a quart glass container or crock, add the sugar to the warm water. Dissolve the yeast in the mixture. Add the flour, stirring well. Let sit in a warm place until fermented and bubbly, 2 to 3 hours. When bubbly and risen a little, cover and refrigerate. Starter is ready to be used. At each using, I find it works best if taken from the refrigerator and allowed to warm about 1 hour before putting into the dough mixture.

After each use, replenish the starter by mixing in ¹/₂ cup lukewarm water and ³/₄ cup rice flour.

SIMPLY SUPER SOURDOUGH

A wonderfully moist and tasty bread that stays fresh for days and is great for sandwiches and toast. If you prefer, you may use three cups of GF flour mix for the separate flours. For the lactose intolerant see Note.

2 cups rice flour
$^1/_2$ cup potato starch flour
$^1/_2$ cup tapioca flour
1 teaspoon salt
$2^1/_2$ teaspoons xanthan
 gum
$1^1/_2$ teaspoons Egg
 Replacer (optional)
$^7/_8$ cup quite warm water
1 teaspoon vinegar or
 $1^1/_2$ teaspoons dough
 enhancer

$^3/_4$ cup sourdough starter
 (page 69)
$^3/_4$ cup cottage cheese
4 tablespoons ($^1/_2$ stick)
 butter or margarine,
 melted
3 eggs, beaten slightly
3 tablespoons sugar
1 tablespoon dry yeast
 granules

Mix together the flours, salt, xanthan gum, and Egg Replacer (if used).

Mix together the water, vinegar, sourdough starter, cottage cheese, butter, and eggs.

Measure the sugar and yeast.

Place the ingredients in the baking pan of the bread maker in the order suggested by your manual. (Some put yeast, then flour, then sugar, then liquids; others suggest the reverse order.)

Bake on regular bread setting on medium heat.

NOTE: For the lactose intolerant change cottage cheese to nondairy sour cream. Reduce water to $^3/_4$ cup.

ITALIAN HERB SOURDOUGH

Another flavorful sourdough. Wonderful with soups and stews. If you'd like, try toasting the dry onion in olive oil for a bit of color. For the lactose intolerant see Note.

1 cup white rice flour
1 cup brown rice flour
1/2 cup potato starch flour
1/2 cup tapioca flour
1/4 cup rice bran
2 1/2 teaspoons xanthan
  gum
1/2 teaspoon salt
1 teaspoon onion salt
1 1/2 teaspoons Egg
  Replacer (optional)
4 teaspoons caraway seeds
1/2 teaspoon fennel seeds
1 to 2 teaspoons dried
  onion
2 teaspoons instant coffee
  powder

3 eggs, beaten
1 teaspoon vinegar or
  1 1/2 teaspoons dough
  enhancer
1/4 cup molasses
3/4 cup sourdough starter
  (page 69)
7/8 cup warm water
3/4 cup cottage cheese
4 tablespoons (1/2 stick)
  butter or margarine,
  melted
1 tablespoon sugar
1 tablespoon dry yeast
  granules

Blend together the flours, rice bran, xanthan gum, salt, onion salt, Egg Replacer (if used), caraway seeds, fennel seeds, onion, and coffee.

Combine the eggs, vinegar, molasses, sourdough starter, water, cottage cheese, and butter.

Measure the sugar and yeast.

Place the ingredients in the baking pan of the bread maker in the order suggested by your manual. (Some add yeast, then flour, then sugar, and then liquids; others suggest the reverse order.)

Bake on regular bread setting on medium heat.

NOTE: For the lactose intolerant change cottage cheese to nondairy sour cream. Reduce water to 3/4 cup.

SANDRA'S MOCK RYE SOURDOUGH

A reader sent in the basis for this recipe, which she developed for her bread machine, for a great-tasting sourdough. Freeze-dried crystals may be used in place of the coffee powder. For the lactose intolerant see Note.

1 cup white rice flour
1 cup brown rice flour
$^1/_2$ cup potato starch flour
$^1/_2$ cup tapioca flour
$^1/_4$ cup rice bran
$2^1/_2$ teaspoons xanthan gum
$1^1/_2$ teaspoons salt
$1^1/_2$ teaspoons Egg Replacer (optional)
4 teaspoons caraway seeds
2 teaspoons instant coffee powder
3 eggs, beaten

1 teaspoons vinegar or $1^1/_2$ teaspoons dough enhancer
$^1/_4$ cup molasses
$^3/_4$ cup sourdough starter (page 69)
$^7/_8$ cup warm water
$^3/_4$ cup cottage cheese
4 tablespoons ($^1/_2$ stick) butter or margarine, melted
1 tablespoon sugar
1 tablespoon dry yeast granules

Blend together the flours, rice bran, xanthan gum, salt, Egg Replacer (if used), caraway seeds, and coffee powder.

Combine the eggs, vinegar, molasses, sourdough starter, water, cottage cheese, and butter.

Measure the sugar and yeast.

Place the ingredients in the baking pan of the bread maker in the order suggested by your manual. (Some put yeast, then flour, then sugar, and then liquids; others suggest the reverse order.)

Bake on regular bread setting on medium heat.

NOTE: For the lactose intolerant change cottage cheese to nondairy sour cream. Reduce water to $^3/_4$ cup.

SHAPED YEAST
BREADS AND ROLLS

ARAB POCKET BREAD
(Pita Bread)

Great! Rounds of flat bread with air-filled pockets for stuffing. Use chicken, ham, or tuna salad fillings and alfalfa or bean sprouts, or try the Gyros filling (page 264). These hand-patted rounds are a bit tricky to make at first but well worth the trouble!

1 cup white or brown rice flour	1/2 cup hot water
2 cups tapioca flour	3 tablespoons shortening
1 cup quick-cooking brown rice cereal (see Note)	1 cup lukewarm water
	1 tablespoon sugar
	2 fresh yeast cakes or
1/2 cup dried milk powder or nondairy substitute	2 tablespoons dried yeast granules
3 teaspoons xanthan gum	1 tablespoon vinegar
1 1/2 teaspoons salt	3 egg whites, room temperature

In the bowl of a heavy-duty mixer, place flours, cereal, dried milk, xanthan gum, and salt.

In the hot water, melt the shortening.

To the lukewarm water add the sugar, then crumble in the yeast. Let stand for a few minutes to foam up.

Using the flat beater on mixer, not the bread hook, blend the dry ingredients on low, then add the hot water and shortening plus the vinegar. Blend. Pour in the yeast mixture and blend again. Add the egg whites; beat on high speed for 4 minutes.

Using a rice-floured board or wax paper, spoon out a dough ball about the size of a goose egg. Use more rice flour if necessary to form a ball you can knead a little. Using as much rice flour as necessary, roll out or hand-pat the dough to a flat circle approximately 4 to 5 inches in diameter, no more than 1/4 inch thick at edges, and slightly thicker in center. Remove to a greased baking sheet dusted with rice flour. Repeat until you have a dozen or so circles.

Cover and let partially rise in a warm place for about 30 minutes. Preheat oven to 500°. Bake sheets, one at a time, for 5 to 6 minutes. Check often to prevent the rounds from becoming too crisp or firm. Remove from sheets to cool.

These may be used immediately, stored in the refrigerator, or frozen. If stored, plump the pockets when ready to use by reheating on high in a microwave for about 25 seconds. If they don't all pop up with a pocket, use a knife to slit one. (Even those from a bakery are not always perfect.) Makes 12 or more pocket loaves.

NOTE: Pacific Rice's Quick 'n Creamy is excellent. Or use Erewhon. If you cannot find brown rice cereal, you may substitute quick-cooking white Cream of Rice.

CRUMPETS
(Lactose and Soy Free)

My favorite bread! One of my testers said this recipe alone would be worth the price of the book. These rich, tender 4-inch buns can be sliced for hamburgers, toasted as English muffins, or filled with ham and cheese for the lunch box. For baking, you will need six English muffin rings, found in most kitchen supply stores. You won't need a heavy mixer; any hand-held electric beater will work. This recipe can be doubled successfully.

1 1/2 cups GF flour mix	1 cup lukewarm water
1 1/2 teaspoons baking powder	1 tablespoon dry yeast granules
1 teaspoon xanthan gum	1 egg, room temperature
1/2 teaspoon salt	1 teaspoon dough enhancer or 1/2 teaspoon vinegar
1 1/2 teaspoons Egg Replacer (optional)	3 tablespoons margarine or butter, melted
1 1/2 tablespoons sugar, divided	

Mix together the flour, baking powder, xanthan gum, salt, and Egg Replacer (if used). Set aside.

Add 1 teaspoon of the sugar to the water and stir in the yeast. Set aside.

Grease 6 English muffin rings and place them on a greased baking sheet.

In a mixing bowl, blend together, using a mixer at low speed, the remaining sugar, egg, margarine, dough enhancer, and yeast water. Beat in half the flour mixture. With a spoon, stir in the remaining flour and beat until smooth.

Pour batter into the prepared rings. Cover and let rise in a warm place until the batter doubles, 40 to 45 minutes for regular yeast; 20 to 25 minutes for rapid rise. Preheat oven to 375°. Bake for 18 to 20 minutes until browned lightly and pulled slightly away from the rings. *Makes 6 crumpets.*

AUSTRALIAN TOASTER BUNS

For those who wish to cut down on egg yolks, use the above recipe but use only 1 egg white and replace the yolk with 1 tablespoon of cottage cheese. *Makes 6 buns.*

GINGER-ORANGE ROLLS

Use these moist muffins with a hint of Malaysia for breakfast (they're quick to stir up in the morning) or for a tasty roll to serve with any Far Eastern dish. If you haven't baked with yeast before, this is an easy recipe for the beginner. You don't need a powerful mixer; any small hand-held electric beater will work.

1 1/2 cups GF flour mix
1 1/2 teaspoons baking
   powder
1 teaspoon xanthan gum
1/2 teaspoon salt
1 tablespoon dry yeast
   granules
1 cup lukewarm water
2 tablespoons sugar
1 whole egg, room
   temperature

1 egg yolk, room
   temperature
4 tablespoons (1/2 stick)
   margarine or butter,
   melted
2 tablespoons fresh grated
   orange rind
1 tablespoon candied
   ginger, chopped

Mix together the flour, baking powder, xanthan gum, and salt. Set aside.

Stir yeast into the water and set aside.

In a large mixing bowl blend, with the mixer at low speed, the sugar, egg and extra egg yolk, margarine, and yeast liquid. Beat in half the flour mixture. With a spoon, stir in the rest of the flour, the orange rind, and ginger. Blend until smooth.

Fill 12 greased muffin cups half full. Cover with a clean dishcloth and let rise in a warm place until the batter doubles, 40 to 45 minutes for regular yeast, 20 to 25 for rapid rise. Preheat oven to 375°. Bake for 18 to 20 minutes until lightly browned and pulled slightly away from pan. *Makes 12 rolls.*

SELF-RISING BREADS

CARAWAY SODA BREAD

The sweet taste of caraway gives a lift to the basic Irish soda bread. This firm, fine-grained bread slices well and is good either hot or cold.

1¹/₂ cups GF flour mix
¹/₂ cup tapioca flour
1¹/₄ teaspoons baking soda
1 teaspoon baking powder
2 teaspoons xanthan gum
¹/₂ teaspoon salt
3 tablespoons sugar

¹/₂ cup (1 stick) butter or
   margarine, softened
1 tablespoon caraway
   seeds
1 cup sour cream
1 tablespoon milk, for
   brushing

Preheat oven to 375°.

Sift flours, soda, baking powder, xanthan gum, salt, and sugar into a large mixing bowl. Cut in butter until the mixture is crumbly. Add caraway seeds and sour cream. Beat with a mixer for about 1 minute, or until well blended.

Form the dough into a round mound in a 7″ greased casserole. Brush with milk. Bake for 50 to 55 minutes. Remove from pan and cool on a wire rack.

If you wish to use this bread sliced thin with appetizer spreads or pâtés, bake it in two 2¹/₂″ × 5″ loaf pans. Cut the baking time by about 10 minutes. Slice when cold. *Makes 1 large round loaf or 2 small loaves.*

AFRICAN SQUASH BREAD

A moist, springy sweet bread so good it may be served as a dessert. If desired, replace the baby food with leftover cooked winter squash. For a special treat make the Cream-filled Squash Gems below.

1³/₄ cups GF flour mix	¹/₂ cup brown sugar
2 teaspoons baking powder	¹/₂ cup (1 stick) margarine
1 teaspoon baking soda	or butter, melted
1¹/₂ teaspoons pumpkin	2 large eggs
pie spice	One 6-ounce jar Junior
1 teaspoon dried orange	baby squash
peel	³/₄ cup plain yogurt
¹/₄ teaspoon salt	¹/₂ cup chopped nuts

Preheat oven to 375°.

In a large mixing bowl, combine flour, baking powder, soda, pumpkin pie spice, orange peel, and salt.

In a smaller bowl, blend together the sugar and butter. Beat in the eggs until smooth. Stir in the squash and yogurt until blended.

Add the liquid mixture and nuts to the dry ingredients. Stir until just moistened. Spoon into three 2¹/₂" × 5" greased and rice-floured pans. Bake for 45 minutes. Cool slightly before removing from pans. Cool thoroughly before slicing. *Makes 3 small loaves.*

For 12 muffins, spoon into 12 large greased muffin cups. Bake for 35 to 40 minutes.

CREAM-FILLED SQUASH GEMS

For an absolutely elegant dessert muffin, use the above recipe but eliminate the nuts. Mix together the following ingredients:

One 3-ounce package cream cheese
1 tablespoon plain yogurt
3 tablespoons sugar

Spoon out only half the dough, dividing it among 12 large greased muffin cups, filling only halfway. Then make a hole in the dough and fill with a spoonful of this filling. Top with the rest of the dough. Bake in a 375° oven for 35 to 40 minutes. *Makes 12 gems.*

CRANBERRY-NUT BREAD

A fruit bread that isn't too sweet; it has a moist texture and a tart taste. The recipe can be modified to eliminate the soy and lactose.

1¹/₂ cups GF flour mix	1 cup brown sugar
¹/₂ cup soy flour	2 eggs
1 teaspoon xanthan gum	1 cup yogurt
¹/₄ teaspoon ground cloves	3 tablespoons butter or
1 teaspoon dried orange	margarine, melted
peel	1 cup fresh or frozen
1 teaspoon salt	cranberries, chopped
2 teaspoons baking powder	¹/₂ cup pecans, chopped
1 teaspoon baking soda	

Preheat oven to 350°.

In a large mixing bowl, blend thoroughly the flours, xanthan gum, cloves, orange peel, salt, baking powder, baking soda, and sugar.

In a smaller bowl, beat the eggs; add the yogurt and butter. Pour this liquid into the flour mixture and stir until blended (don't beat). Stir in the cranberries and nuts.

Pour into one 5″ × 8″ greased and rice-floured loaf pan or into three 2¹/₂″ × 5″ prepared loaf pans. Bake 60 to 65 minutes for a large loaf, or 35 to 40 minutes for small loaves. Cool thoroughly before slicing. *Makes 1 large or 3 small loaves.*

FOR THE SOY OR LACTOSE INTOLERANT: Omit the soy flour and orange peel. Replace the yogurt with ³/₄ cup orange juice. The texture is not as good, but the flavor is delicious.

ENGLISH TEA SCONES
(with Devonshire Cream)

My mouth had been watering for these ever since a trip to Devon when I had to eat my rice cake while others were downing their scones with cream and jam. Success came after years of failure. These are tender, chewy, and flavorful. Use them for your fruit shortcakes, too.

1 cup white rice flour	2 tablespoons brown sugar
1/2 cup tapioca flour	1/4 cup (1/2 stick) butter or
2 teaspoons baking powder	margarine
1 teaspoon baking soda	1/2 cup (approximately)
1/2 teaspoon xanthan gum	plain yogurt
2 tablespoons white sugar	

Preheat oven to 400°.

In a medium mixing bowl, blend together the flours, baking powder, baking soda, xanthan gum, and sugars. Add the butter and cut with fork (or rub with your fingers) until the mixture resembles coarse meal.

Stir in as much of the yogurt as you need for the dough to form a soft ball. Place this on a rice-floured board and knead slightly. Roll out the dough to 3/4 inch thick. Cut into rounds with a 2 1/2-inch cookie cutter and place the rounds on a greased baking sheet. Bake for 10 to 12 minutes. *Makes 10 to 12 scones.*

Top with Devonshire Cream and a dollop of fruit jam.

DEVONSHIRE CREAM

Blend 1 tablespoon confectioner's sugar and 1 teaspoon vanilla into 1 cup cultured sour cream. The cream can be prepared ahead and chilled for several days. *Makes 1 cup cream.*

FRENCH CREAM

Substitute 1/2 cup cottage cheese for half of the sour cream. Then prepare this topping like Devonshire Cream, above, but add a bit more confectioner's sugar and $^1/_8$ teaspoon nutmeg with the vanilla. Blend in a blender or food processor.

GRATED APPLE LOAF

A moist, sweet bread that is as American as apple pie and great for brunch, tea, or snacking. It keeps well because of the moisture from the fruit and soy flour.

$^3/_4$ cup soy flour
$^1/_2$ cup potato starch flour
$^1/_4$ cup rice flour
$^3/_4$ teaspoon baking soda
1 teaspoon baking powder
$1^1/_4$ teaspoons cream of tartar
$^1/_2$ teaspoon xanthan gum (optional)
1 teaspoon grated lemon peel

1 teaspoon cinnamon
$^1/_4$ teaspoon nutmeg
$^1/_4$ teaspoon allspice
$^1/_2$ teaspoon salt
$^1/_3$ cup shortening
$^2/_3$ cup sugar
2 eggs, well beaten
$^3/_4$ cup grated apple
$^1/_2$ cup chopped nuts (optional)

Preheat oven to 350°.

Sift the flours, soda, baking powder, cream of tartar, xanthan gum (if used), lemon peel, cinnamon, nutmeg, allspice, and salt together. Set aside.

In a large mixing bowl, cream the shortening. Gradually add the sugar, beating until light and fluffy. Add the eggs and beat again. Add the flour alternately with the grated apple, a small amount at a time, beating after each addition until smooth. Stir in the nuts (if used). Pour into a well-greased and rice-floured 5″ × 9″ loaf pan. Bake for 1 hour. For doneness, test with toothpick. It should come out clean. *Makes 1 loaf.*

ALMOND-CHEESE BREAD

A wonderful idea from England, this bread stays moist for days, probably because of the tomato sauce used as the liquid—which no one ever suspects when they exclaim over the great taste.

1½ cups GF flour mix
1 teaspoon baking soda
1 rounded teaspoon baking powder
½ teaspoon xanthan or guar gum
½ teaspoon salt
½ cup shortening

½ cup sugar
3 eggs
One 8-ounce can tomato sauce
⅔ cup grated Cheddar cheese
½ cup sliced almonds

Preheat oven to 350°.

Sift together the flour, baking soda, baking powder, xanthan gum, and salt. Set aside.

In a large mixing bowl, cream the shortening and sugar. Add the eggs, one at a time, beating after each addition. Stir in the flour mixture until just mixed. Add the tomato sauce, cheese, and almonds. Mix well, but don't beat.

Pour into a greased 5″ × 8″ loaf pan. Bake for 40 to 45 minutes or until a toothpick comes out clean. For easy removal, cool 10 minutes in the pan.

Makes 1 loaf.

ALMOND-CHEESE MUFFINS: Fill greased muffin pans ¾ full. Bake for 20 to 25 minutes. *Makes 18 muffins.*

FRUIT AND
FIBER MUFFINS

A crunchy, high-fiber muffin so tasty it can almost be a dessert. Vary the fruit, nuts, vegetable, and even the cereal—and have a taste from a different country with each change. For example, use banana instead of kiwifruit, shred zucchini or apple for the carrot, and use any nut you choose. If you don't have brown rice cereal, substitute Cream of Rice. The xanthan gum is optional, but without it the muffin will be more crumbly.

1 cup brown rice flour	1/2 cup raisins
1/4 cup brown rice cereal	1/2 cup (2 kiwis) mashed
1/2 teaspoon xanthan gum	kiwifruit
(optional)	1/2 cup shredded carrot
1 1/2 teaspoons baking	1/2 cup chopped nuts
powder	2 eggs
3/4 teaspoon baking soda	1/4 cup milk or nondairy
1 teaspoon dried orange	liquid
peel	2 tablespoons vegetable oil
1/2 cup brown sugar	

Preheat oven to 400°.

In a large mixing bowl, blend together the flour, cereal, xanthan gum (if used), baking powder, soda, orange peel, and sugar.

Cover the raisins with very hot water and let soak while you prepare the kiwifruit, carrots, and nuts.

In a small bowl, beat the eggs slightly. Add the milk and oil. Pour into the dry ingredients and stir until just blended. The batter will be lumpy.

Drain the raisins and add along with the kiwifruit, carrot, and nuts to the flour mixture. Stir until blended. Pour the batter into greased muffin tins and bake for 15 to 18 minutes or until a toothpick comes out clean. Let set for a few minutes in the tins to finish cooking before removing. *Makes 12 muffins.*

KIWI MUFFINS

The blend of exotic taste and delicate, springy texture of these muffins makes them my favorite fruit bread. You may change the kiwi to banana and the carrot to zucchini, if necessary, but you will lose some of the flavor that makes these so good.

1¼ cups GF flour mix
½ teaspoon xanthan gum
1½ teaspoons baking powder
¾ teaspoon baking soda
½ teaspoon salt
1 teaspoon dried orange peel
⅓ cup brown sugar
2 eggs

¼ cup milk or nondairy liquid
2 tablespoons margarine or butter, melted
½ cup (2 kiwis) mashed kiwifruit
½ cup shredded carrot
½ cup chopped cashew nuts

Preheat oven to 400°.

In a large mixing bowl, blend together the flour, xanthan gum, baking powder, baking soda, salt, orange peel, and sugar.

In a small bowl, beat the eggs slightly. Add the milk and margarine. Pour this mixture into the dry ingredients and stir until just blended. The batter will be lumpy.

Add the kiwifruit, carrot, and nuts. Stir until blended.

Pour into greased muffin tins and bake for 15 to 18 minutes until browned slightly. Let set a few minutes in the tins to finish cooking before removing. *Makes 12 muffins.*

SWEDISH HARDTACK

Firm, flat rounds that taste great, keep well, and are perfect for traveling. Good with cheese, sliced meat, or just plain. Carry some in a plastic bag in a purse or a pocket for eating when others will be served cookies or crackers. Use either fresh buttermilk or powdered buttermilk prepared with water.

2¹/₂ cups brown rice flour
1 tablespoon xanthan gum
1 teaspoon baking soda
1 teaspoon salt
2 teaspoons dried orange
   peel

2 cups buttermilk
¹/₂ cup dark brown sugar
¹/₂ cup (1 stick) butter or
   margarine, melted

Preheat oven to 425°.

In a medium bowl, blend together the flour, xanthan gum, baking soda, salt, and orange peel. Set aside.

In a large mixing bowl, stir together the buttermilk, sugar, and butter. Add half the flour mix and beat with a spoon to a smooth batter. Stir in the remaining flour to form a thick dough. (You may have to add a bit more flour. Humidity and the thickness of the buttermilk will make a difference—I use powdered and make it richer than the box suggests.)

Pick up small portions of the dough and, using your hands, roll into 1-inch balls. Add more flour, if necessary. With your hands, flatten these balls to the thickness of pie dough and into circles 2¹/₂ or 3 inches in diameter. Place on an ungreased baking sheet and prick all over with a fork before baking.

Bake for 8 to 10 minutes, turning once if they are browning too much on one side. After all the biscuits are baked, pile them together on one baking sheet and return to the oven. *Turn off oven* and let them sit for 5 to 6 hours (or overnight).

If they are not crisp enough, reheat the oven, turn it off, and put the hardtack back for another 2 hours. Store in airtight containers for up to a month. To keep longer, freeze. *Makes 6 dozen 2¹/₂- to 3-inch crackers.*

FLAKY BREAKFAST RUSKS

Crisp, buttery flavored rusks that keep well for traveling. Pack these in a plastic container and enjoy your own continental breakfast while your companions are eating their gluten pastry. Vary the flavor by substituting dried orange peel or cardamom, or use some brown rice flour in the GF flour mix.

1²/₃ cups GF flour mix	1 teaspoon dried lemon
¹/₃ cup sweet rice flour	peel
1¹/₂ teaspoons xanthan	¹/₄ teaspoon salt
gum	²/₃ cup margarine or butter
4¹/₂ teaspoons baking	1 egg
powder	¹/₂ cup nondairy liquid,
2 teaspoons Egg Replacer	unthinned*
(optional)	1 teaspoon dough enhancer
1¹/₂ teaspoons sugar	(optional)

Preheat oven to 425°. Grease two 12″ × 16″ baking sheets.

In a large mixing bowl, combine flours, xanthan gum, baking powder, Egg Replacer (if used), sugar, lemon peel, and salt. Add cold margarine in small chunks. Cut in with a pastry blender until coarse crumbs form.

In a small bowl, beat egg, nondairy liquid, and dough enhancer (if used). Add to the flour mixture and stir quickly into a smooth, firm dough ball.

Split ball in half and form a loaf about ¹/₂ inch thick and 3 inches wide. Cut crosswise into 8 even pieces and place on one greased baking sheet. Repeat with second half of dough. Bake in oven for about 10 minutes or until lightly browned. Remove and reduce oven temperature to 250°.

Cool the rusks slightly and split in half. Return to the cooler oven and bake about 25 minutes or until crisp. Turn the oven off and let it cool completely before removing rusks. Store at room temperature in closed containers for up to one month. *Makes 32 rusks.*

*If allergic to soy, replace the nondairy liquid with thin cream or half-and-half.

MOCK GRAHAM CRACKERS

All the flavor and wholesomeness of real graham crackers. This easy, no-fail cracker keeps well in a closed container, is a good traveler, and is a tasty substitute for cookies. The crackers are also great for pie crust (page 148). For added flavor, sprinkle cinnamon sugar on some before baking.

³/₄ cup (1¹/₂ sticks) butter
   or margarine
¹/₄ cup honey
1 cup brown sugar
1 teaspoon vanilla
1¹/₂ cups brown rice flour
1¹/₂ cups GF flour mix

2 tablespoons soy flour
1 teaspoon xanthan gum
1 teaspoon salt
1 teaspoon cinnamon
3 teaspoons baking powder
¹/₂ to ³/₄ cup water

Preheat oven to 325°.

In a large mixing bowl, beat together the butter, honey, sugar, and vanilla.

In another bowl, blend together the flours, xanthan gum, salt, cinnamon, and baking powder. Stir this into the creamed mixture alternately with the water, using just enough water to hold the batter in a soft ball. Refrigerate for at least 1 hour.

Roll out half the dough on a brown rice–floured piece of plastic wrap to a rectangle about ¹/₂ inch thick. Transfer to a greased 12″ × 15¹/₂″ baking sheet by putting the pan over the dough, holding the wrap, and flipping. Continue to roll out the dough until it covers the sheet and is about ¹/₈ inch thick. Trim the edges. Cut with a pastry wheel into 3-inch squares. Prick each square 5 times with a fork.

Bake for about 30 minutes, removing the crackers around the edges if they get too brown.

Repeat with the other half of the dough. *Makes 40 crackers.*

BREAKFAST BREADS

DROP SCONES
(Scotch Pancakes)

A delicious pancake so thick and bready it can be split and filled with jam, egg, or bacon for a breakfast muffin. It stays firm and can also be stuffed like pita bread for lunch. Both the method of mixing and the flavor are unusual. Make ahead and warm in the microwave for an easy breakfast bread—a gluten-free "McMuffin."

1 cup GF flour mix	1 teaspoon dark corn
1/3 teaspoon xanthan gum	syrup
1 egg, beaten	2 tablespoons butter or
1/2 cup milk or nondairy	margarine, melted
liquid	2 teaspoons baking powder
2 1/2 tablespoons sugar	1/4 teaspoon salt

In a medium mixing bowl, blend the flour and xanthan gum. Add the egg and then beat into the flour mixture, gradually adding the milk. Beat to the consistency of thick cream.

Add the sugar, syrup, butter, baking powder, and salt. Beat well.

Drop the batter onto a medium-hot Teflon or lightly greased griddle by the tablespoon to make scones 2 1/2 inches in diameter. Cook as for any pancake, but since these are thicker, they will need to be on the heat longer, so don't have the griddle extra hot, or you will have doughy centers. Serve hot. Split to fill with butter and jam, sausage, or cheese. *Makes 5 to 6 scones.*

RAISED DOUGHNUTS

After years of trying, I finally succeeded in creating a raised doughnut that tastes like those I think I remember. My nonceliac tasters didn't guess that these were made without gluten flour. Make a double batch, for they will go fast either hot or cold. You may shake these in sugar, as I suggest, or frost for a fancier treat.

1¹/₂ cups GF flour mix	1 cup lukewarm water
2 tablespoons soy flour	1 tablespoon rapid-rise dry
1¹/₂ teaspoons baking	yeast granules
powder	3 tablespoons margarine,
1 teaspoon xanthan gum	melted
¹/₂ teaspoon salt	2 eggs, room temperature
1 teaspoon apple pie	1 quart vegetable oil
spice	3 to 4 tablespoons sugar,
¹/₃ cup sugar, divided	for dusting

Blend the GF flour mix, soy flour, baking powder, xanthan gum, salt, and spice. Set aside.

Add 1 teaspoon of the sugar to the water and then stir in the yeast. Set aside until it foams slightly.

In a large mixing bowl, blend together with a hand mixer at low speed the remaining sugar, the margarine, eggs, and yeast mixture. Beat in half the flour mix. Stir in the rest of the flour and beat with a spoon until smooth.

Heat oil to 370° in an electric frying pan or a deep fryer.

Place the dough in a doughnut maker (see Note) and press out onto hot oil, 3 or so at a time. (If the dough becomes too thick to press out of the maker, stir in 1 tablespoon of warm water at a time until it drops out easily.) Turn once to brown on both sides. Remove with tongs and drain on paper toweling.

While still warm, shake in a plastic bag with sugar.

If you prefer to frost, wait until cool and frost with a simple confectioner's sugar or one of the icings from pages 119–20. *Makes 2 dozen 2¹/₂-inch doughnuts.*

NOTE: A doughnut maker is a press like a cookie press and can be purchased inexpensively at kitchen supply shops and some hardware stores. If you don't have a press, use the recipe above, cutting the egg to 1 egg plus 1 egg yolk and adding 2 or more tablespoons of rice flour in order to make a slightly thicker dough; press the dough from a plastic bag with a 1/2-inch slit cut at a corner. Press the shape of a circle over the hot fat. These may be slightly lopsided or not closed but they taste just as delicious.

BAKED DOUGHNUTS

A boon for those who are trying to avoid deep-fried foods, these may come out slightly flat on one side, but the flavor is excellent warm or cold.

Use the Raised Doughnuts recipe but eliminate the oil for frying and use 3 tablespoons of margarine or butter, melted, for brushing. Instead of frying in the deep fat, press the batter onto greased cookie sheets. Brush the doughnuts with melted margarine (fingers work best here). Cover and let rise in a warm place until doubled in size, approximately 20 minutes.

Bake in a preheated 425° oven for 10 to 12 minutes, or until the doughnuts are slightly browned. (I turn on the broiler for about 1 minute at the end to complete browning.)

While still hot, brush again with melted margarine. Dust with sugar, as above, or frost as desired.

FRUITED BREAKFAST TORTE

A fruited combination of a Dutch Baby and a pancake that is easy to make and sure to be a hit at any breakfast or brunch.

4 tablespoons (¹/₂ stick)
  butter or margarine
4 eggs, beaten
³/₄ cup whole milk or
  nondairy liquid
³/₄ cup GF flour mix

¹/₄ teaspoon salt
¹/₄ cup brown sugar
2 tablespoons lemon juice
1 cup thinly sliced fresh
  fruit (apples, papaya,
  peach, etc.; see Note)

Preheat oven to 425°.

Melt the butter and pour it into a 9″ pie pan.

Combine the eggs, milk, flour, and salt until just blended. Pour into the butter in the pie pan.

Add the sugar and lemon juice to the fruit and tumble until the slices are coated. Place the sugared pieces on top of the batter, either at random or in a spoke pattern. Bake for 15 minutes. Cut into wedges and serve immediately. You may top with a dollop of whipped cream, ice cream, or yogurt, if desired. *Serves 4.*

NOTE: If using apples, after tumbling them with the sugar and lemon juice, microwave them for 3 to 4 minutes to precook them before placing on the torte.

CAKES

LAYER CAKES

Black Forest Cake
Yellow Velvet Cake
Lemon Torte

BUNDT AND ANGEL FOOD CAKES

Chocolate-Applesauce Bundt
   Cake
Pacific Rim Cake
Zucchini Bundt Cake
Chocolate Mist Angel Food
Curaçao Orange Bundt
   Cake
Hawaiian Isles Chiffon Cake

SHEET CAKES

Gingerbread
Scandinavian Spice Cake

Chinese Five-Spice Cake
Danish Spice Cake with
   Crumb Topping

CAKES WITH FILLINGS OR SAUCES

Sacher Torte
Double Dutch Treat
Clafoutis
Sponge Roll
   Jelly Roll
   Lemon Roll
   Ice Cream Roll
   Ice Cream Cake

CHEESECAKES

White Chocolate Cheesecake
Black Forest Cheesecake
Ricotta-Pineapple Cheesecake

FILLINGS, FROSTINGS, AND SAUCES

Mock Cherry Filling

Lemon Filling

Coconut-Pecan Frosting

Baker's Secret Icing

Mocha Cream Frosting

Lemon Sauce

Orange Sauce

How many times have you attended (or given) a party where the centerpiece was a lovely, decorated, gluten-filled cake? Frustrating, isn't it, when you can't eat it, as no birthday or wedding is complete without its centerpiece of decorated cake?

After experimenting with many recipes, I have converted some of the most popular American and foreign cakes to our safe flours. In other recipes in this section I have used spices, fruits, chocolate, and seasoning from around the world to create the taste of other lands.

Most of your friends probably pick up a mix from the wide choice on the grocery shelf (or order from a bakery) when they want a cake. For us, it takes a bit more time—but not much. And you, too, can have a choice of some wonderfully moist, great-flavored cakes to serve at that next party.

In recipes calling for sour cream, if you are soy intolerant, use cultured sour cream but decrease the amount of flour by 1/4 cup.

For many of the recipes, I use my own formula for a flour mix. You may purchase my GF flour mix from a supplier (see page 343) or mix it yourself. The formula is:

> 2 parts white rice flour
> 2/3 part potato starch flour
> 1/3 part tapioca flour

LAYER CAKES

BLACK FOREST CAKE

An absolutely wonderful meld of chocolate and cherries. My nonceliac tasters agree that this, even with the substitute flours, is the real thing. For filling, use the recipe below or use Mock Cherry Filling (page 118).

The cake crumbs when dried and crushed are wonderful as crumbs for Rum Balls (page 135), for the crumb crust for any of the cheesecakes (pages 115 to 117) or for the bottom crust of the Four-Layer Dessert (page 174).

Cake

2¹/₄ cups GF flour mix
1 teaspoon xanthan gum
2 teaspoons baking soda
¹/₂ teaspoon salt
¹/₂ cup (1 stick) margarine
  or butter
2 cups brown sugar
3 eggs
3 squares semisweet
  chocolate, melted
1¹/₂ teaspoons almond
  flavoring
1 cup plain yogurt
1 cup cherry cola, regular
  cola, or other
  carbonated soft drink

Filling

One 17-ounce can pitted
  dark cherries
¹/₄ cup sugar
1 tablespoon cornstarch
1 tablespoon tapioca flour

1 recipe Baker's Secret
  Icing (page 120)
Sweet chocolate (optional)
5 maraschino cherries
  (optional)

Preheat oven to 350°.

In a medium bowl, sift together the flour, xanthan gum, baking soda, and salt. Set aside.

In a large mixing bowl, cream together the margarine and sugar until light and fluffy. Add the eggs, one at a time. Add the chocolate and flavoring. Add the dry ingredients alternately with the yogurt, beating well after each addition.

Heat the cola to boiling and stir into the batter, which will make it quite thin. Pour into 2 greased and rice-floured 8″ cake pans. Bake for 35 to 45 minutes, or until the tester comes out clean. Cool in pans for 10 minutes and then remove to cool on wire racks.

While the cake is cooling, prepare the cherry filling: Drain the cherries, pouring the juice into a small saucepan. Put the juice over medium heat. In a small bowl, mix together the sugar, cornstarch, and tapioca flour. Blend in a few spoonfuls of the hot juice until you have a thin paste. Pour this into the remaining juice and cook a few minutes until thickened slightly. Remove from heat. Use as much of the thickened juice as you need to mix with the cherries for a spreadable filling.

To put the cake together, be sure the top of the bottom layer is level. You may have to cut off the rounded top. Spread a thick layer of cherry filling; add the top cake layer. Anchor with toothpicks. Frost with Baker's Secret Icing. To make this look authentic, you may use shaved sweet chocolate around the outside and decorate with maraschino cherries on top. Enjoy!

YELLOW VELVET CAKE

A fine-textured, great-flavored, moist yellow cake. Use this as the base for your favorite layer cakes, or cut the recipe in half for a simple dessert served with fruit and whipped cream or ice cream, or make it into a Lemon Torte with the filling on the next page.

2¼ cups GF flour mix	1 teaspoon salt
3 teaspoons baking powder	4 eggs
1 teaspoon baking soda	1⅓ cups sugar
1 teaspoon xanthan gum	⅔ cup mayonnaise
2 teaspoons dried lemon peel	1 cup 7UP (Diet okay)

Preheat oven to 350°.

In a medium bowl, blend together the flour, baking powder, baking soda, xanthan gum, lemon peel, and salt. Set aside.

In a large mixing bowl, beat together the eggs, sugar, and mayonnaise until fluffy and lemon colored. Add the flour mixture alternately with the 7UP, beating with a spoon after each addition.

Spread the batter into 2 greased and rice-floured 8″ or 9″ round cake pans or into a greased and rice-floured 9″ × 13″ oblong pan. Bake for 25 to 30 minutes for round cake, slightly more for the oblong cake. The top will spring back when done. Frost or fill with any of your favorite icings.

LEMON TORTE

Lemon Torte is easy to assemble but impressive! My tasters wouldn't believe it was gluten free. This can be made a day ahead for a party; it keeps well.

1 recipe Yellow Velvet
  Cake (page 97)
1 recipe Baker's Secret
  Icing (page 120)
One 14-ounce can
  sweetened condensed
  milk

1/2 cup lemon juice
2 teaspoons fresh grated
  lemon rind
Yellow food coloring

Prepare Yellow Velvet Cake using 2 round pans.

In a medium bowl, beat together the milk, lemon juice, lemon rind, and a few drops of the food coloring. Set in the refrigerator to thicken as it chills.

Split each cake layer into 2 layers either by cutting with a knife or using a thread. Spread the filling (using 1/4 each time) completely over each of the first 3 layers. For the top layer, spread the filling to 1 inch from the outside edge.

Frost the sides and the bare inch around the top with the Baker's Secret Icing. Chill for at least 2 hours. *This rich torte will make 12 to 16 servings.*

BUNDT AND
ANGEL FOOD CAKES

CHOCOLATE-APPLESAUCE
BUNDT CAKE

This rich, moist chocolate cake, filled with nuts and raisins, needs no frosting. It keeps well wrapped in plastic and stored in the refrigerator and is even better the second day, when flavors have mingled.

2 cups GF flour mix	1¹/₃ cups brown sugar
1 teaspoon xanthan gum	3 eggs
1¹/₂ teaspoons baking powder	1¹/₃ cups applesauce
1¹/₂ teaspoons baking soda	1¹/₂ tablespoons lemon juice
¹/₂ teaspoon salt	²/₃ cup chopped walnuts
2 teaspoons pumpkin pie spice	²/₃ cup raisins
1 teaspoon Egg Replacer (optional)	1¹/₂ teaspoons grated lemon rind
²/₃ cup mayonnaise	2 squares semisweet baking chocolate, melted

Preheat oven to 350°.

Sift together the flour, xanthan gum, baking powder, baking soda, salt, spice, and Egg Replacer (if used). Set aside.

In a large mixing bowl, beat the mayonnaise and sugar until light and fluffy. Add eggs, one at a time, beating constantly. Stir in the applesauce and lemon juice. Add the flour, except for ¹/₄ cup.

Toss the reserved flour with the nuts, raisins, and lemon rind.

Add the chocolate and then the floured nut mixture to the batter.

Pour into a greased and rice-floured 3-quart bundt pan and bake 50 minutes. Test for doneness by inserting a toothpick in the cake. It should come out clean.

Remove from the oven and invert the pan to let the cake cool before unmolding.

PACIFIC RIM CAKE

A moist, tender bundt cake, rich with the flavors of the Pacific Rim nations. It needs only a thin lime icing drizzled on while still warm to make it complete. This cake keeps well if wrapped in plastic and seems to have more flavor the second day.

2¹/₂ cups GF flour mix
1 teaspoon xanthan gum
1¹/₂ cups sugar
1¹/₂ teaspoons baking soda
2 teaspoons baking powder
1 teaspoon Egg Replacer
 (optional)
1 teaspoon salt
2 teaspoons dried orange
 peel
¹/₂ teaspoon nutmeg
¹/₂ teaspoon cloves
³/₄ cup mayonnaise
¹/₃ cup milk or nondairy
 liquid

3 eggs, beaten slightly
4 kiwifruit, mashed
 (about 1¹/₃ cups)
¹/₂ cup toasted almonds or
 macadamia nuts,
 chopped (see Note)
3 tablespoons candied
 ginger, minced

Lime Icing

1 cup confectioner's sugar
3 tablespoons hot lime
 juice

Preheat oven to 350°.

In a large mixing bowl, place flour, xanthan gum, sugar, baking soda, baking powder, Egg Replacer (if used), salt, orange peel, nutmeg, and cloves. Blend with a mixer on low.

Add the mayonnaise, milk, and eggs. Beat until well mixed. The dough will be thick. Beat in the kiwifruit until well blended and smooth. Stir in the chopped nuts and minced ginger.

Pour into a well-greased and rice-floured 3-quart bundt pan. Bake for 50 to 55 minutes, or until the top springs back when lightly pressed. Remove from the oven, let stand for about 5 minutes, and then invert onto a large cake plate or round of cardboard covered with foil.

While the cake is still hot, combine the icing ingredients and drizzle them on the cake.

NOTE: To toast nuts, spread them in a single layer in a shallow pan. Bake at 300° to 325° about 10 minutes, stirring often. The nutmeats will change from ivory to tan and will continue to toast slightly after they have been removed from the oven.

ZUCCHINI BUNDT CAKE

Zucchini rises to new heights in this moist and tender cake, which needs only a drizzled glaze of confectioner's sugar mixed with a little orange or lime juice for completion. It keeps moist for days.

2 cups white rice flour	1 teaspoon dried lemon
1 cup tapioca flour	peel
1 teaspoon xanthan gum	4 eggs
2 teaspoons Egg Replacer	1¹/₂ cups sugar
(optional)	1 cup mayonnaise
¹/₂ teaspoon salt	3 cups grated zucchini
3 teaspoons baking powder	1 cup finely chopped
1¹/₂ teaspoons baking soda	walnuts
1¹/₂ teaspoons apple pie	Frosting of choice or Lime
spice	Icing (page 100)

Preheat oven to 350°.

In a medium bowl combine flours, xanthan gum, Egg Replacer (if used), salt, baking powder, baking soda, apple pie spice, and lemon peel. Blend thoroughly.

In a large mixing bowl, beat the eggs, sugar, and mayonnaise until light. Fold in the zucchini.

Add the nuts to the flour mixture. Stir them into the batter until just blended. Pour the batter into a greased and rice-floured 3-quart bundt pan. Bake 1 hour and 15 minutes, or until tester comes out clean.

Cool for 10 minutes in the pan, then invert onto a cake plate or round of cardboard covered with foil.

Cake may be frosted, if desired, or (as I prefer) drizzled, while still hot, with a thin glaze of icing prepared with lime or orange juice.

CHOCOLATE MIST
ANGEL FOOD

This angel-light cake has a blush of chocolate and is easy to make.

1/2 cup confectioner's sugar
1/4 cup potato starch flour
1/4 cup cornstarch
2 tablespoons cocoa
   powder
1/3 cup granulated sugar
7 egg whites (3/4 cup),
   room temperature

3/4 teaspoon cream of
   tartar
1/4 teaspoon salt
1 teaspoon almond or
   vanilla flavoring

Preheat oven 375°.

Sift together the confectioner's sugar, flour, cornstarch, and cocoa powder. (The sifting is essential in this recipe.)

Measure the granulated sugar to have handy.

In a large glass or metal (not plastic) mixing bowl, place the egg whites, cream of tartar, salt, and flavoring. Blend with a mixer at high speed and, continuing to beat, slowly add the granulated sugar. Beat until the sugar is dissolved and the whites form stiff peaks.

With a rubber spatula, gently fold in the flour mixture (about 1/4 at a time), folding just enough so the flour mixture disappears. Pour the batter into an ungreased 9″ tube pan and cut through with a table knife to break any air bubbles. Bake for 35 minutes, or until the top springs back after being lightly pressed. Invert pan to cool. Remove only when completely cool.

Recipe can be doubled for large 10″ tube pan.

CURAÇAO ORANGE BUNDT CAKE

This moist cake, rich with the flavors of the Caribbean island of Curaçao, keeps well and needs no frosting except for the simple orange-rum glaze drizzled on while still warm.

Grated rind of 1 lime
2 tablespoons rum
2 cups GF flour mix
1½ teaspoons baking powder
1 teaspoon baking soda
1 teaspoon xanthan gum
½ teaspoon salt
⅔ cup mayonnaise
1⅓ cups sugar
3 eggs

¼ cup orange juice
1 teaspoon dried orange peel
⅔ cup buttermilk

Glaze

½ cup orange juice
½ cup sugar
1 tablespoon rum (optional)

Preheat oven to 350°.

In a small bowl, place the lime zest and rum.

In a medium bowl, sift together the flour, baking powder, baking soda, xanthan gum, and salt.

In a mixing bowl, combine the mayonnaise and sugar. Beat until blended. Add the eggs, orange juice, orange peel, and rum–lime zest mixture. Beat a few seconds. Add the buttermilk and beat again. With a spoon, fold in the flour mixture, one-third at a time until blended. Pour into a greased and rice-floured 10″ bundt pan.

Bake for 45 to 50 minutes, or until the top springs back after being lightly pressed. Let stand for about 10 minutes while making the glaze. Then loosen the cake using a thin spatula and invert it onto a rack.

To make the glaze: In a medium saucepan heat the orange juice and sugar until sugar dissolves. Add the rum and cook for 8 to 10 minutes, or until the mixture is syrupy. Drizzle this, while still hot, over the cake, letting it soak in.

HAWAIIAN ISLES CHIFFON CAKE

Tender and flavored with tropical fruits and coconut. This cake needs no frosting except a light icing of confectioner's sugar blended with butter and tropical fruit juice. Or top it with a lemon or orange sauce (see page 121 or 122).

2 cups GF flour mix	One 6-ounce can
1¹/₂ cups sugar	pineapple-orange-banana
1 tablespoon baking	juice (³/₄ cup)
powder	1 teaspoon dried lemon peel
1 teaspoon salt	¹/₂ teaspoon cream of
¹/₂ cup vegetable oil	tartar
7 eggs, separated	1 cup dried coconut

Preheat oven to 325° for a tube pan, to 350° for an oblong pan.

In a large mixing bowl, blend together the flour, sugar, baking powder, and salt. Make a well in this mixture and add, in order, the oil, unbeaten egg yolks, fruit juice, and lemon peel. Beat with a spoon until smooth.

In a large metal bowl, beat with an electric mixer the egg whites and cream of tartar until they form very stiff peaks.

Add the coconut to the egg yolk mixture and pour it gradually over the whipped whites, gently folding with a rubber scraper until just blended.

Pour batter into a large ungreased tube pan or a 9″ × 13″ oblong pan. Bake the tube cake in a 325° oven for 55 minutes, then raise the heat to 350° for 10 to 15 minutes. Bake the oblong cake in a 350° oven for 45 to 50 minutes, or until the top springs back after being lightly pressed.

SHEET CAKES

GINGERBREAD

This hearty dessert cake was brought to America by northern Europeans.

2¹/₄ cups GF flour mix
2 teaspoons ginger
2 teaspoons cinnamon
²/₃ teaspoon cloves
1 teaspoon baking soda
²/₃ cup sugar
¹/₂ teaspoon salt
3 eggs

²/₃ cup light molasses
²/₃ cup nondairy sour
  cream substitute (see
  Note)
²/₃ cup mayonnaise
Whipped cream, Lemon
  Sauce (page 121), or
  Orange Sauce (page 122)

Preheat oven to 350°.

In the bowl of a mixer, blend together the flour, ginger, cinnamon, cloves, baking soda, sugar, and salt.

In a smaller bowl, beat the eggs; add the molasses, sour cream substitute, and mayonnaise. Pour the liquid into the dry ingredients and beat at medium speed for 1 minute (do not overbeat).

Pour the batter into a greased and rice-floured 8″ × 8″ pan. Bake for 40 to 45 minutes, or until the cake top cracks and a tester comes out clean. Let the cake cool in the pan.

Serve hot or cold with whipped cream, or, for a contrasting taste, try topping the cake with Orange Sauce or Lemon Sauce.

NOTE: If soy intolerant use cultured sour cream but decrease the amount of flour by ¹/₄ cup.

SCANDINAVIAN SPICE CAKE

A delicate, tender spice cake that can be eaten either hot or cold with a simple topping of whipped cream. If you want to dress it up, frost with Mocha Cream Frosting or Baker's Secret Icing.

1¹/4 cups GF flour mix
  (see Note)
2 teaspoons baking powder
¹/2 teaspoon baking soda
¹/2 teaspoon xanthan gum
2 large eggs
²/3 cup sugar
2 teaspoons cinnamon
1 teaspoon ginger
1 teaspoon cloves

¹/2 teaspoon salt
¹/3 cup mayonnaise
²/3 cup nondairy sour
  cream substitute
  (see Note)

Whipped cream, Mocha
  Cream Frosting (page
  120), or Baker's Secret
  Icing (page 120)

Preheat oven to 350°.

Sift together the flour, baking powder, baking soda, and xanthan gum. Set aside.

In a large mixing bowl, beat the eggs and sugar until light and foamy. Stir in the cinnamon, ginger, cloves, and salt. Add the flour mixture, stirring only until smooth.

Stir in the mayonnaise and sour cream substitute until well blended (do not beat). Pour the batter into a greased and rice-floured 8″ × 8″ pan. Bake for 30 to 35 minutes, or until the top springs back after being lightly pressed and the sides pull slightly away from the pan. Serve hot or cold with whipped cream, or cool the cake before frosting with Mocha Cream Frosting or Baker's Secret Icing.

NOTE: If soy intolerant use cultured sour cream but decrease the amount of flour by ¹/4 cup. This recipe may be doubled for a 9″ × 13″ pan.

CHINESE FIVE-SPICE CAKE

Exotic spices and fruit from the East Indies plus a lemon icing spread on while the cake is still hot give this dessert an excitingly different taste and an explosion of flavor! It is so good that I had to hide it when testing to see if it would stay moist. It does. Crushed, drained, unsweetened pineapple may be substituted for the kiwifruit, but the flavor will not be as exotic.

Cake

2¹/₄ cups GF flour mix (see Note)

1 teaspoon xanthan gum

4 teaspoons Chinese-style five-spice seasoning (see Note)

3 teaspoons baking soda

¹/₂ teaspoon salt

¹/₂ cup Butter Flavor Crisco

1¹/₂ cups brown sugar

4 eggs

1¹/₂ teaspoons dried lemon peel

1¹/₂ cups plain yogurt

1 cup kiwifruit (about 4 to 5) peeled and mashed

Icing

1¹/₂ cups confectioner's sugar

3 tablespoons hot lemon juice

1¹/₂ tablespoons minced sugared ginger

Whipped cream or ice cream (optional)

Preheat oven to 350°.

In a medium bowl, combine flour, xanthan gum, five-spice seasoning, baking soda, and salt. Set aside.

In a large mixing bowl, cream the Crisco and sugar until light and fluffy. Beat in the eggs and lemon peel. Add the dry ingredients alternately with the yogurt, beating after each addition (do not overbeat). Stir in the kiwifruit.

Pour the batter into a greased and rice-floured 9″ × 12″ baking pan. Bake for 35 to 45 minutes, or until a tester inserted into the center comes out clean. Let set 5 minutes and, with a large kitchen fork, poke holes into the top of the cake.

Icing: in a bowl combine the sugar, lemon juice, and ginger. Spread the icing over the cake while still hot.

Serve as is in squares or with a scoop of whipped cream on top. It is also excellent with ice cream.

NOTE: This cake can easily be halved. Just use one-half of all cake ingredients and bake in an 8″ × 8″ pan. Shorten the baking time to 25 to 30 minutes. For the icing, use two-thirds of ingredient quantities.

Chinese-style five-spice seasoning is a mixture of spices including fennel, anise, ginger, licorice root, cinnamon, and cloves. It can be found in the spice or oriental section of grocery stores and in oriental markets.

DANISH SPICE CAKE WITH CRUMB TOPPING

A fellow celiac in Seattle shares this easy old family recipe with a few changes to our flours and additives. Any leftovers of this richly flavored cake are wonderful, dried and crushed, for crumb crusts for pies or cheesecakes. For the lactose intolerant, see Note.

1 scant cup GF flour mix
    or rice flour
3/4 cup sweet rice flour
1 teaspoon baking soda
1 teaspoon Egg Replacer
    (optional)
1/2 teaspoon xanthan gum
1 1/2 teaspoons cinnamon
1 teaspoon cloves
1/4 teaspoon allspice
1 cup sugar
1/4 teaspoon salt
1/2 cup shortening
1 egg

2 tablespoons molasses
1 cup sour milk or
    buttermilk

Topping

2 tablespoons butter,
    melted
1 tablespoon sweet rice
    flour
4 tablespoons sugar
1/2 teaspoon cinnamon
1/4 cup chopped almonds
    (optional)

Preheat oven to 350°.

In a mixing bowl, sift together the flours, baking soda, Egg Replacer (if used), xanthan gum, cinnamon, cloves, allspice, sugar, and salt. Cut in the shortening until a fine crumb texture is obtained.

Add the egg and molasses to the flour mixture. Blend well using a hand mixer. Add the sour milk and beat until the batter is smooth. Pour into a well-greased 8″ × 8″ pan.

Topping mix: Melt the butter. Add the flour, sugar, cinnamon, and almonds (if used). Mix and then crumble over the top of the batter. Bake for 45 to 50 minutes or until the top springs back when lightly touched.

NOTE: For the lactose intolerant, mix 1/2 cup nondairy sour cream with 1/2 cup nondairy liquid, or, if you can tolerate yogurt, use yogurt, thinning it by using 1/3 part nondairy liquid.

CAKES WITH FILLINGS
OR SAUCES

SACHER TORTE

On my first visit to Europe many years ago, I was told there are three things a tourist must do in Vienna: view the Lippizan horses, attend the opera, and, afterward, order Sacher torte at the famous Sacher Hotel. The opera was dramatic, the horses magnificent, and the Sacher torte out of this world, with a lovely layer of jelled apricot on the bottom.

When I got home, I tried to make a cake that tasted like that Sacher torte; after a lot of experimenting (and failures), I felt I had the flavor. Then, as a celiac, I had to start all over with our safe flours. Finally, using a chocolate cake as a base, here is my version of Sacher torte that you can enjoy without packing your suitcase.

1¹/₂ cups GF flour mix
¹/₂ teaspoon xanthan gum
1 teaspoon baking soda
¹/₄ teaspoon salt
¹/₄ cup (¹/₂ stick)
    margarine or butter
1 cup dark brown sugar
2 small eggs
1¹/₂ squares semisweet
    chocolate
¹/₂ cup plain yogurt

¹/₂ cup cola drink
³/₄ cup apricot jam

One 16-ounce can GF
    fudge frosting (see Note)
    or Mocha Cream
    Frosting (page 120)
Whipped cream (optional)
Chocolate shavings
    (optional)

Preheat oven to 350°.

In a small bowl, sift together the flour, xanthan gum, baking soda, and salt.

In a mixing bowl, cream together the margarine and sugar until light and fluffy. Beat in the eggs, one at a time.

Melt the chocolate and add it to the creamed mixture.

Add the dry ingredients alternately with the yogurt, beating well after each addition.

Heat the cola to boiling and stir it into the batter, which will make it quite thin. Pour into a greased 8″ or 9″ square pan. Drizzle the jam over the batter, letting it sink in.

Bake for about 40 minutes, or until a tester inserted in center comes out clean. Cool in pan before frosting.

Ice with fudge frosting and then, to serve most authentically, cut into squares and top with whipped cream and shaved chocolate. Or, for a less rich dessert, ice only with Mocha Cream Frosting and serve. *Makes 9 servings.*

NOTE: Gluten-free fudge frostings are available in grocery stores.

DOUBLE DUTCH TREAT

A real treat for the chocoholic, this quick and easy chocolate cake is baked in its own rich, fudgy sauce. Double Dutch Treat can be stirred up and put in the oven at the same time you cook your dinner. Serve plain, hot or cold, or with a topping of ice cream or whipped cream.

Batter

1 cup GF flour mix
1/2 teaspoon xanthan gum
2 teaspoons baking powder
1/4 teaspoon salt
3/4 cup granulated sugar
2 tablespoons cocoa
2 tablespoons butter or
  margarine, melted
1/2 cup milk or nondairy
  liquid
1 teaspoon vanilla

1/2 cup chopped nuts
  (walnuts or pecans)

Sauce

1 cup brown sugar
1/4 cup cocoa powder
1 3/4 cups cola, heated to
  boiling, or 1 2/3 cups hot
  coffee plus 2 tablespoons
  rum
Ice cream or whipped
  cream (optional)

Preheat oven to 350°.

Batter: In a large mixing bowl, sift together the flour, xanthan gum, baking powder, salt, sugar, and 2 tablespoons cocoa.

In a small bowl, combine the butter, milk, and vanilla. Add this mixture to the dry ingredients and blend until mixed. Stir in the nuts. Spread the batter in a greased 8″ square pan.

Sauce: Combine the sugar and cocoa. Sprinkle the mixture over the batter. Pour the cola gently over the batter.

Bake in oven for 45 to 55 minutes until the cake top springs back when touched lightly. Serve with a scoop of ice cream or a dollop of whipped cream (if desired). *Makes 6 to 8 servings.*

CLAFOUTIS

This French upside-down cobbler is an easy dessert especially good when fresh fruit is in season. Make it with peaches, apples, or rhubarb, but cherries are traditional. Serve warm or cold with a dollop of whipped cream or a scoop of ice cream or frozen yogurt.

Sauce

2 tablespoons butter or margarine
2 cups fresh fruit, washed or peeled, pitted, and sliced
1 tablespoon lemon juice
2 tablespoons water
1/2 cup plus 2 tablespoons sugar

Batter

1 cup plus 2 tablespoons GF flour mix
1 1/2 teaspoons baking powder
1/2 teaspoon baking soda
1/2 teaspoon xanthan gum
1/2 cup plus 2 tablespoons sugar
2 eggs
1/3 cup mayonnaise
1 teaspoon dried lemon peel
1/2 teaspoon salt
7UP or plain yogurt
Whipped cream, ice cream, or frozen yogurt (optional)

Preheat oven to 350°.

Sauce: In a small saucepan, melt the butter. Add the fruit, lemon juice, water, and sugar. (If using rhubarb, omit the lemon and add an extra tablespoonful of sugar; if using apples, add $^{1}/_2$ teaspoon of cinnamon.) Cook for about 5 minutes over medium heat. Then drain the juice into a cup measure and allow the remaining fruit to cool while making the batter.

Batter: In a small bowl blend the flour, baking powder, baking soda, and xanthan gum.

In a medium mixing bowl, beat together the sugar, eggs, mayonnaise, lemon peel, and salt until they are light. Beat in the flour mixture.

Add enough 7UP or yogurt to the reserved juice to make $^{1}/_2$ cup. Beat the mixture into the batter.

Pour the batter into a greased 8″ square pan. Drop the sauce in dollops onto the batter.

Bake for about 45 minutes, or until a tester inserted in the center comes out clean. *Makes 6 generous servings.*

SPONGE ROLL

One of my treasures from the past altered to be gluten free sounds a bit complicated, but once you've tried it, you'll find it easy to make. The basic sponge cake can be rolled and filled with jelly, a fruit or lemon filling, or ice cream to create many different desserts. Another use is as ladyfingers for the Down-Under Trifle on page 176.

4 large eggs, room temperature	1 teaspoon dried lemon peel
$^{1}/_2$ cup rice flour	$^{2}/_3$ cup sugar
$^{1}/_4$ cup tapioca flour	$^{1}/_2$ teaspoon cream of tartar
$^{1}/_4$ cup teaspoon salt	Confectioner's sugar
1 teaspoon baking powder	

Preheat oven to 375°.

Prepare a 9″ × 13″ pan by lining the bottom with wax paper and lightly greasing it.

Separate the eggs, yolks into a small bowl, whites into a large one.

In another small bowl, blend together the rice flour, tapioca flour, salt, baking powder, and dried lemon peel. Set aside.

Beat the egg yolks until thick and lemon colored. Set aside.

Beat the egg whites for 1 minute, then add 1 tablespoon of the sugar and the cream of tartar. Continue beating until the whites are glossy and stiff, 4 to 5 minutes. Remove the beater.

With a spoon, gently fold the egg yolks into the whites. Fold in the rest of the sugar in 3 parts, then the dry ingredients. Pour the batter into the prepared pan and bake for 18 to 20 minutes, or until the top springs back after being lightly pressed. Immediately invert onto a smooth cotton tea towel dusted with confectioner's sugar. Carefully remove the wax paper. Immediately roll the sponge cake and tea towel. Let cool. Unroll and spread with desired filling. Roll up again (without the towel) and dust the top with confectioner's sugar; wrap with wax paper. To serve, cut into 1-to-1½-inch slices. *Makes 6 to 8 servings.*

JELLY ROLL: Thin your favorite jelly or jam with a little fruit juice to a spreading consistency and spread on the cake before rolling.

LEMON ROLL: Spread the cake with Lemon Filling (page 119) before rolling.

ICE CREAM ROLL: Spread the cake with softened GF ice cream. Roll, dust with confectioner's sugar, wrap in aluminum foil, and place in the freezer. Remove the roll 10 minutes before cutting into slices for serving.

ICE CREAM CAKE: Instead of rolling, cool the cake flat on the towel and then cut into 3 sections (each 9 by 4.33 inches). Cut 1 quart of GF brick ice cream (vanilla is always good, but your favorite can be used) into ½-inch slices. Place a section of cake on a large piece of aluminum foil, add a layer of ice cream, then another section of cake and another layer of ice cream. Top with cake. Frost top and sides with 1 cup of whipped cream sweetened to taste and colored (if desired) with food coloring. Tent a 16-by-12-inch piece of foil and seal it around the cake without touching the frosting and place in the freezer. Remove from the freezer 10 minutes before serving. Cut into 1-inch slices. *Makes 8 servings.*

CHEESECAKES

WHITE CHOCOLATE CHEESECAKE

This make-ahead cake is absolutely sinful. The combination of chocolate and cheese raises the simple cheesecake to gourmet heights. If the cake or cookie crumbs are not chocolate, you must add dried cocoa.

Crust

1¹/₂ cups dried chocolate cake or cookie crumbs
1 tablespoon cocoa powder (if crumbs are not chocolate)
2¹/₂ tablespoons margarine or butter, melted

Filling

1 cup cottage cheese
One 8-ounce package cream cheese, softened
3 eggs
²/₃ cup sugar
1 tablespoon lemon juice
2 tablespoons rice flour
3 squares white baking chocolate, melted

Preheat oven to 375°.

Crust: Tumble together the crumbs, cocoa (if using), and butter. Pat into the bottom of a 9″ pie plate or 8″ springform pan, reserving 2 tablespoons for sprinkling on top (if desired).

Filling: Whip cottage cheese in a blender or mixer until smooth and creamy. Add the cream cheese, eggs, sugar, lemon juice, and flour. Beat thoroughly. Stir in the chocolate. Pour into the crust and scatter on the reserved crumbs (if desired). Bake for 35 to 40 minutes, or until set.

Refrigerate for several hours before serving. *Serves 8 to 10.*

BLACK FOREST CHEESECAKE

An easy-to-make, eye-appealing, and delicious cheesecake with all the flavors of the cake from which it takes its name. If the cake or cookie crumbs are not chocolate, add dried cocoa.

Crust

1¹/₂ cup dried chocolate
    cake or cookie crumbs
1 tablespoon cocoa powder
    (if crumbs are not
    chocolate)
3 tablespoons butter or
    margarine, melted

Cake

Two 8-ounce packages
    cream cheese, softened

1 cup cottage cheese
4 eggs
1 cup sugar
1 tablespoon cherry-
    flavored brandy (kirsch)
¹/₂ cup semisweet
    chocolate chips
¹/₂ cup maraschino
    cherries, drained and
    chopped

Preheat oven to 375°.

Combine the crumbs, cocoa (if using), and butter. Pat into a 10″ springform pan.

In a large mixing bowl, beat together the cream cheese, cottage cheese, eggs, and sugar until well blended and smooth. Stir in the brandy, chocolate chips, and cherries. Pour gently into the crust. Bake for 35 to 40 minutes, or until the center is set.

When cool, refrigerate for several hours, or overnight, before serving. *This rich cake can serve 12.*

RICOTTA-PINEAPPLE CHEESECAKE

A fruited cheesecake with fewer calories than the preceding ones. Crushed GF cereal plus 1 tablespoon of sugar may replace the cookie crumbs in the crust.

Crust

1¼ cups GF cookie
  crumbs
¼ cup ground almonds
3 tablespoons margarine or
  butter, melted

Filling

3 eggs, separated
One 15-ounce container
  ricotta cheese

⅔ cup sugar
2 tablespoons cornstarch
1 teaspoon dried orange
  peel
One 8½-ounce can
  crushed pineapple,
  drained

Preheat oven to 375°.

Crust: Mix together the crumbs, nuts, and margarine. Pat into an 8″ springform pan or a 9″ pie plate.

Filling: Beat the egg whites until stiff but not dry. In a large bowl, beat together the ricotta cheese, egg yolks, sugar, cornstarch, and orange peel. Stir in the pineapple. Gently fold in the beaten egg whites. Pour into the crust. Bake for approximately 40 minutes, or until a knife inserted in the center comes out clean. Serve warm or cool. *Makes 8 servings.*

FILLINGS, FROSTINGS, AND SAUCES

MOCK CHERRY FILLING

A great filling for your Black Forest Cake (page 96). Make this ahead and you'll have enough for several cakes. Use up those green tomatoes or firm tomatoes at the supermarket; really ripe tomatoes don't work.

2¹/2 cups green tomatoes (2 to 3 tomatoes)	1 tablespoon lemon juice
2 cups sugar	One 3-ounce box black cherry gelatin
Dash salt	

Peel and quarter the tomatoes. Remove and discard the section of seeds. Mash or dice the remaining soft parts; cut the firm outer casings into thin strips about 1 inch long and 1/4 inch wide. (These will resemble cherries in the finished filling.)

In a 2¹/2-quart saucepan, combine the tomatoes with the sugar and salt. Bring to a boil and cook for 10 minutes, stirring frequently. Remove from heat.

Add the lemon juice and stir in the gelatin. Return to heat and bring to a boil, stirring constantly. Boil for 1 minute. Cool slightly and put in cup-sized containers; refrigerate for up to a month. For keeping longer, put in freezer containers and freeze. *Makes 3 cups (enough for 3 cake fillings).*

LEMON FILLING

This is an easy, light filling for a two-layer cake or for Sponge Roll (page 113). Double the recipe if you wish to fill a three-layer cake.

3/4 cup sugar
3 tablespoons cornstarch
1/2 teaspoon salt
3/4 cup water
1 tablespoon butter or
  margarine

2 tablespoons grated lemon
  rind
1/3 cup lemon juice

In a 1-quart saucepan, combine the sugar, cornstarch, and salt, blending thoroughly. Add the water and bring to a boil. Boil for 1 minute. Remove from heat and add butter, lemon rind, and lemon juice. Let cool before spreading on cake. *Makes 1 cup (enough for covering 1 cake layer or 1 sponge roll).*

COCONUT-PECAN FROSTING

This frosting can sometimes be found gluten free in the market, but beware! I have noticed that two brands contain gluten, so this is a GF recipe. It makes a large batch but keeps well for a week in the refrigerator and months in the freezer. This is most easily made with a mixer that has a heavy-duty beater.

3/4 cup evaporated milk
1 cup sugar
3 eggs, beaten
1/3 cup butter or margarine

1 teaspoon vanilla
1 1/4 cups flaked coconut
1 cup pecans, chopped

In a saucepan, combine the milk, sugar, eggs, and butter. Cook over low heat, stirring constantly, until mixture thickens. Remove from heat and, using a mixer, beat in the vanilla, coconut, and pecans until the frosting is of spreading consistency. *Makes 3 cups.*

BAKER'S SECRET ICING

Have you ever wondered what's in those creamy white icings on the cakes in the bakery? Wonder no more. This is an easy-to-make, never-fail, fluffy white icing. Better yet, it keeps your cake moist.

2 tablespoons sweet rice flour	1 cup sugar
2 tablespoons cornstarch	1 cup vegetable shortening (see Note)
1 cup milk or nondairy liquid	1 teaspoon salt
	1 teaspoon vanilla

In a small saucepan, place the flour and cornstarch. Add a bit of the milk to form a paste, then stir in the rest. Cook over medium heat, stirring constantly, until the paste is thick. Set aside to cool completely (you may put it in the refrigerator).

In a medium bowl, whip together the sugar and shortening, then add the salt and vanilla. Blend in the milk paste. Beat hard until the icing is fluffy. *Makes about 2¹/₂ cups of icing.*

NOTE: Use white shortening for a white frosting, Butter Flavor Crisco for a creamy off-white one, which makes a fine topping for spice and ginger cakes.

MOCHA CREAM FROSTING

A melt-in-your-mouth coffee-chocolate frosting to fill or top any cake, it's easy to make since it requires no cooking.

1 cup margarine or butter, softened	1 teaspoon almond flavoring
2 squares semisweet chocolate, melted	2 cups confectioner's sugar
2 teaspoons freeze-dried coffee	

In a medium sized bowl, blend together the butter and chocolate using a hand mixer. Add the coffee and almond flavoring; blend again. Add the sugar 1/2 cup at a time, beating after each addition. Beat until light and fluffy, a couple of minutes. *Makes approximately 2 cups.*

LEMON SAUCE

A tangy sauce to serve hot over gingerbread or to spice up leftover cake. This sauce keeps well for up to a week in the refrigerator. Reheat to serve.

1/2 cup sugar	2 tablespoons lemon juice
1 tablespoon cornstarch	1 teaspoon dried lemon
1 cup boiling water	peel
1 tablespoon butter or	
margarine	

In a small saucepan, blend together the sugar and cornstarch. Stir in the boiling water, butter, lemon juice, and lemon peel. Bring back to a boil and simmer until thickened, 5 or 6 minutes. *Makes 1 cup.*

ORANGE SAUCE

For angel food cake or hot gingerbread, this rich sauce is a good way to use up leftover egg yolks. It will keep for several days if refrigerated.

3 egg yolks	3/4 cup orange juice
1 teaspoon dried orange	1/2 cup sugar
rind	1/2 cup whipped cream or
1/4 teaspoon salt	nondairy substitute

Combine egg yolks, orange rind, salt, orange juice and sugar in top of a double boiler. Cook over hot water until thickened enough to coat spoon. Remove from heat and chill. Fold in the whipped cream. *Makes about 1 1/4 cups.*

COOKIES

DROP COOKIES

Paradise Drops
Oatmeal Cookies (Mock)
Christmas Fruit Mounds
Nutty Pumpkin Treats
Granola Cookies
Sesame Dollars
   Almond Dollars

BAR COOKIES

Regency Bars
Shortbread
Mediterranean Fruit Bars

SHAPED COOKIES

Rum Balls
Almond-Rice Cookies
Chinese Gingers
Almond-Orange Biscotti
   Almond Biscotti
   Licorice Biscotti
   Christmas Biscotti
   Chocolate-topped Biscotti
Lebkuchen (German Honey
   Cakes)
   Mary's Lebkuchen Balls
Chocolate Surprise Rounds
Crescent Crisps

We call them cookies; to the English and Australians, they're biscuits; and in China, some cookies are known as dot hearts. Call them what you will, cookies are popular with children—and to the child in all of us.

Making cookies is the easiest of all gluten-free baking and seldom requires the use of xanthan gum; so why not keep the cookie jar full of a selection from this wide assortment of flavors from around the world?

Some of the recipes in this section call for rice or soy flour; some, for leftover cake or cookie crumbs; others use a mixture of flours called GF flour mix. This can be purchased from suppliers (see page 343) or you can mix your own. The formula is:

> 2 parts white rice flour
> 2/3 part potato starch flour
> 1/3 part tapioca starch

DROP COOKIES

PARADISE DROPS

Macadamia nuts, coconut, and white chocolate combine to make this taste of paradise. Easy to make, the drops are impossible to keep unless you hide them.

$^1/_2$ cup (1 stick) butter or
  margarine
$^1/_4$ cup granulated sugar
$^1/_3$ cup dark brown sugar
1 large egg
1 teaspoon vanilla
$^3/_4$ cup rice flour
$^1/_2$ cup soy flour
$^1/_2$ teaspoon baking soda

$^1/_2$ teaspoon baking
  powder
Dash salt
$^1/_2$ cup macadamia nuts,
  chopped coarsely
6 ounces white chocolate
  chips
$^1/_2$ cup shredded coconut

Preheat oven to 375°.

In a large mixing bowl, beat the butter, granulated sugar, brown sugar, egg, and vanilla until fluffy.

In a separate bowl, blend the rice flour, soy flour, baking soda, baking powder, and salt. Add to the butter mixture, stirring until well blended. Fold in the nuts, chocolate chips, and coconut. The dough will be very stiff.

Drop by rounded teaspoonfuls onto lightly greased cookie sheets. Bake for about 10 minutes, or until lightly browned. Remove from tin and cool. Store in an airtight container. *Makes 3$^1/_2$ to 4 dozen 1$^1/_2$-inch cookies.*

OATMEAL COOKIES (MOCK)

If you've been hungering for the chewy texture and nutty flavor of oatmeal cookies even since your doctor eliminated gluten from your diet, this is the recipe for you. The almonds, which replace oats, can be purchased in bulk at larger grocery stores or in some discount markets.

1 cup Butter Flavor Crisco	1/2 cup white rice flour
1 cup granulated sugar	1/2 teaspoon salt
1 cup brown sugar	1 teaspoon baking soda
2 eggs	3 cups thin-shaved
1 teaspoon vanilla	almonds (crushed to
1 cup sweet rice flour	oatmeal size; see Note)

Preheat oven to 350°.

In a large mixing bowl, cream together the shortening, granulated sugar, and brown sugar. Beat in the eggs, one at a time. Add the vanilla.

In a separate bowl, blend together the flours, salt, and baking soda. Stir into the creamed mixture. Add the almonds. Drop by rounded teaspoonfuls onto a greased cookie sheet and bake for 10 minutes, or until lightly browned. Remove from pan immediately and cool flat on wax paper. *Makes 6 1/2 dozen 2 1/2-inch cookies.*

NOTE: Place the sliced almonds in a plastic bag and, using a rolling pin, crush to a texture resembling oats.

CHRISTMAS FRUIT MOUNDS

The flavor of this tender, delicate fruited cookie is a change from the usual spicy taste of desserts containing candied fruits. The cookies' shape, taste, and easy preparation make them a great addition to a Christmas tray.

$^1/_2$ cup ricotta cheese
$^1/_2$ cup (1 stick) butter or margarine, softened
1 cup brown sugar
1 egg
$^1/_2$ teaspoon vanilla extract
$^1/_4$ teaspoon dried lemon peel
1$^1/_2$ cups GF flour mix, divided

$^1/_2$ teaspoon baking soda
$^1/_2$ teaspoon baking powder
$^1/_2$ teaspoon salt
$^1/_2$ cup chopped candied fruit
$^1/_2$ cup dried currants or golden raisins
Candied cherries, halved, for decoration (optional)

Preheat oven to 375°.

In a large mixing bowl, blend the cheese and butter. Cream in the sugar. Add the egg, vanilla, and lemon peel, and beat until light and fluffy.

In a separate bowl, sift together the flour, baking soda, baking powder, and salt. Add all but $^1/_2$ cup to the batter. Stir thoroughly. Mix the candied fruit and raisins into the remaining flour, and add to the batter.

Drop by rounded teaspoonfuls onto greased cookie sheets, leaving 2 inches between drops. If desired, center a cherry half on each cookie. Bake for 8 to 10 minutes, or until slightly browned. *Makes 4$^1/_2$ dozen cookies.*

NUTTY PUMPKIN TREATS

A moist and flavorful blend of pumpkin, spices, raisins, and nuts, these are easy to make, and they keep and travel well. This recipe can easily be doubled.

$^1/_2$ cup (1 stick) butter or margarine
1 cup brown sugar
1 cup cooked pumpkin
1 teaspoon vanilla
1 cup rice flour
1 cup soy flour
1 teaspoon baking soda

1 teaspoon baking powder
$^1/_2$ teaspoon salt
$^1/_2$ teaspoon cinnamon
$^1/_2$ teaspoon nutmeg
$^1/_4$ teaspoon ginger
$^1/_4$ teaspoon allspice
1 cup golden raisins
$^1/_2$ cup chopped pecans

Preheat oven to 350°.

In a large mixing bowl, beat together the butter and sugar. Add the pumpkin and vanilla. Beat until well mixed.

In a separate bowl, blend together the rice flour, soy flour, baking soda, baking powder, salt, cinnamon, nutmeg, ginger, and allspice. Stir into the pumpkin mixture until smooth. Stir in the raisins and nuts. Drop by teaspoonfuls onto lightly greased baking sheets and bake 12 to 15 minutes, or until lightly browned. *Makes 4$^1/_2$ dozen cookies.*

GRANOLA COOKIES

A tasty, crunchy drop cookie, easy to make. This is not so sweet that it will spoil appetites. But it is satisfying, travels well, and keeps its flavor when stored in a closed container.

1¹/₂ cups rice flour
¹/₂ cup soy flour
1 teaspoon baking soda
1 teaspoon baking powder
¹/₂ cup (1 stick) butter or margarine, room temperature

1 cup brown sugar
1 egg
1 teaspoon vanilla
3 tablespoons plain yogurt
2¹/₂ cups granola (page 189), chopped or ground in food processor

Preheat oven to 375°.

Blend together the flours, baking soda, and baking powder. Set aside.

In a large mixing bowl, cream the butter and sugar using an electric mixer. Add the egg, vanilla, yogurt, and blend. Add the flour mixture and beat until smooth.

With a spoon, stir in the granola. Drop by rounded teaspoonfuls onto greased cookie sheets and bake for 10 to 12 minutes, or until lightly browned. *Makes 4 dozen cookies.*

SESAME DOLLARS

Sesame is one of the oldest food plants known to man. Three thousand years ago the Egyptians ground the seeds into flour. Today, tahini, a paste made of the seeds, is used in many Mediterranean dishes. These thin, chewy, dollar-shaped cookies make use of tahini, found in most large food stores. Flavorful and crispy, these are great travelers.

2 eggs	1 cup brown or granulated
2 teaspoons Egg Replacer	sugar
(optional)	1 teaspoon salt (if tahini is
1 cup tahini	unsalted)

Preheat oven to 350°.

In a medium bowl, beat the eggs and Egg Replacer (if used). Stir in the tahini, sugar, and salt (if used).

Drop by small teaspoonfuls onto ungreased cookie sheet and bake for 10 to 12 minutes, or until lightly browned. Remove immediately from pan to cool. *Makes about 4 dozen 1½-inch cookies.*

ALMOND DOLLARS: Replace the tahini with almond butter, found in most large grocery stores in the section with peanut butter and jams.

BAR COOKIES

REGENCY BARS

A frosted bar baked with its own topping, created originally for the Swedish royal family. Even with our flours, it's a royal taste treat.

Base

1/2 cup (1 stick) margarine
   or butter
1/2 cup sugar
2 egg yolks
1 drop almond oil or
   1 teaspoon almond
   flavoring
3/4 cup sweet rice flour

1/2 cup white rice flour
1/2 teaspoon salt
1 teaspoon baking powder

Topping

2 egg whites
1/2 cup sugar
4 ounces almond paste

Preheat oven to 350°.

Base: Cream the margarine and sugar. Beat in the egg yolks, then the almond oil.

Sift together the flours, salt, and baking powder; add to the creamed mixture.

Pat the base into an 8″ × 8″ baking pan and bake for 25 minutes. While baking, make the topping.

Topping: Whip the egg whites until stiff, adding the sugar a little at a time. Blend in the almond paste and beat until smooth. Spread over the baked base and return to the oven for about 18 to 20 minutes, or until the topping is firm. Cool before cutting into 1-by-1 1/2-inch bars. *Makes about 3 dozen small bars.*

SHORTBREAD

This very easy recipe was carried to America by a young Scottish emigrant who came here as an au pair girl. The granddaughter of her "family" says this shortbread tastes as good as the original even when converted to our gluten-free flour.

$^{1}/_{2}$ cup (1 stick) butter or
   margarine, softened
4 tablespoons cornstarch

$^{1}/_{4}$ cup sugar
$^{1}/_{2}$ cup sweet rice flour

Preheat oven to 325°.

Place the butter in a medium mixing bowl. Sift the cornstarch and sugar over it and work in. Add the sweet rice flour and work until the dough feels plastic.

Spoon into an 8″ × 8″ pan and pat down, using a little flour on fingers so they won't stick to the dough. Prick the sheet of dough liberally with a fork. Bake for 12 minutes, or until the batter starts to turn golden. Cut immediately into 1$^{1}/_{4}$-by-1$^{1}/_{4}$-inch squares. Let cool in pan before removing. *Makes 3 dozen squares.*

MEDITERRANEAN FRUIT BARS

These flavorful, fruited treats, with variations for sugar- and egg-free versions, can serve from a lunch box cookie to a dinner dessert (when topped with a dab of whipped cream).

2/3 cup dates, chopped
2/3 cup dried apricots, chopped
2/3 cup golden raisins
1 tablespoon lemon juice
1 cup water
1/4 cup margarine or butter
1 cup GF flour mix
2 tablespoons soy flour
1/2 teaspoon xanthan gum
1 teaspoon baking soda
1 teaspoon dried orange peel

1/4 teaspoon salt
1/2 teaspoon cinnamon
1/4 teaspoon nutmeg
1/4 teaspoon cloves
2 tablespoons brown sugar or 1 teaspoon liquid sugar substitute
2 eggs, beaten, or 1/2 cup Egg Beaters
1/2 cup chopped walnuts

Preheat oven to 350°.

In a medium saucepan, combine dates, apricots, raisins, lemon juice, and water. Simmer 5 minutes, stirring occasionally. Stir in margarine and set aside to cool.

In a large mixing bowl, blend together the flour mix, soy flour, xanthan gum, baking soda, orange peel, salt, cinnamon, nutmeg, cloves, and brown sugar. (If using liquid sugar, add it later.) Stir in the fruit mixture and eggs (and liquid sugar, if used) until well blended. Add the nuts.

Spread the batter in a greased 9″ × 13″ baking pan and bake for 15 to 20 minutes or until top springs back when touched lightly. Cool before cutting into 1-by-2-inch bars. *Makes 4 1/2 dozen bars.*

SHAPED COOKIES

RUM BALLS

An easy no-bake cookie. Rum gives a touch of the Caribbean to the American bourbon ball. This recipe can use up your GF cake or cookie leftovers (or failures).

2¹/₂ cups GF cake or
   cookie crumbs
1 cup confectioner's sugar
1 cup finely chopped
   walnuts
2 tablespoons unsweetened
   baking chocolate, melted

¹/₄ to ¹/₃ cup dark rum
4 to 5 tablespoons corn
   syrup
Extra confectioner's sugar,
   for rolling finished balls

Whirl the crumbs in a food processor until fine, or dry them thoroughly and crush with a rolling pin.

In a medium mixing bowl, blend the crumbs, sugar, and walnuts. Add the chocolate and rum. Stir well and add about 3 tablespoons of the corn syrup. Add more as needed in order to make the dough stick together enough to form ³/₄-inch balls.

Roll balls in confectioner's sugar and chill for at least 12 hours, allowing the flavors to blend. These keep well in an airtight container. *Makes approximately 5 dozen balls.*

ALMOND-RICE COOKIES

Although the Chinese do not serve desserts often, these almond-flavored cookies might accompany a dish of cooked apricots or mandarin oranges at the end of a banquet.

1 cup white rice flour	6 tablespoons peanut oil
3/4 cup confectioner's sugar	1 egg, well beaten
1/4 teaspoon salt	1 teaspoon almond
1/2 cup finely ground	flavoring
almonds	Whole blanched almonds

Preheat oven to 375°.

In a mixing bowl, blend together flour, sugar, salt, and almonds. Add the peanut oil and cut the dough using a fork until it feels like cornmeal. Stir in the egg and flavoring. This should form a dough that will roll out on a lightly rice-floured board.

Roll about 1/4 inch thick. Cut cookies into small 1 3/4-to-2-inch rounds and press a whole blanched almond in the center of each. Remove to a greased cookie sheet and bake for 15 minutes. *Makes twenty-four 2-inch cookies.*

CHINESE GINGERS

This spicy ginger cookie is very different from the preceding mild, almond-flavored rice cookie. If you like the flavor of ginger, try this for your next oriental dinner.

1 cup (2 sticks) butter or	1/4 teaspoon Chinese-style
margarine	five-spice seasoning
3/4 cup brown sugar	(see Note)
1/4 cup minced candied	1 1/2 cups rice flour
ginger	1/2 cup tapioca flour
2 teaspoons vanilla	1/4 cup granulated sugar,
	for dipping

Preheat oven to 375°.

In a mixing bowl, cream together the butter and brown sugar. Add the candied ginger and vanilla.

In a separate bowl, blend together the five-spice seasoning and two flours. Gradually add this mixture to the creamed mixture to form a stiff dough.

Roll the dough into 1-inch balls, dipping half of each into water and then into sugar to coat. Shake each ball and then place sugar side up on an ungreased cookie sheet. Bake for 10 to 12 minutes, or until slightly brown. Let stand for 5 minutes before removing to cool on a wire rack. Handle carefully, for these crumble easily until cool. Store in an airtight container. These cookies will keep up to 3 weeks in a closed container. *Makes about 4 dozen cookies.*

NOTE: Chinese-style five-spice seasoning can be purchased in most supermarkets or food specialty shops.

ALMOND-ORANGE BISCOTTI

Twice-baked for a crunchy texture and a sticklike shape, these cookies are well worth the extra time. Everyone loves them, for they're not sweet, can serve as bread or a sweet snack, and are great with coffee or wine. And, they keep well. The xanthan gum is optional, but, without it, the cookies will tend to crumble.

1 cup slivered almonds	3 cups GF flour mix
3/4 cup sugar	4 teaspoons baking powder
1/2 cup (1 stick) butter or margarine	2 1/2 teaspoons dried orange peel
1/3 cup white corn syrup	1 1/2 teaspoons xanthan gum (optional)
1 teaspoon vanilla	
4 eggs	

Preheat oven to 350°.

Place the almonds in an 8″ square pan and bake until lightly toasted, 8 to 10 minutes. Let cool, then chop coarsely and set aside.

In a large mixing bowl, beat together the sugar, butter, corn syrup, and vanilla until smooth. Add eggs, one at a time, beating after each addition.

In a separate bowl, mix together the flour, baking powder, orange peel, and xanthan gum (if used). Add to the egg mixture, stirring to blend. Add the chopped almonds.

Grease 2 cookie sheets. Spoon the dough into 4 flat loaves on the sheets; each loaf should be about 1/2 inch thick, 2 inches wide, and the length of the cookie sheet. Bake for about 25 minutes (reversing the position of the sheets halfway through the baking). When done the loaves should be browned at the edges and springy to the touch.

Let the loaves stand on the cookie sheets until cool to touch. Cut diagonally into slices 1/2-inch thick. Arrange slices on their sides on the baking sheets and return to the oven to bake again until the cookies are brown and crisp, 15 to 18 minutes (again, reverse the position of the pans halfway through baking).

After cooling, the *biscotti* can be stored in an airtight container for up to a month. *Makes about 4 dozen* biscotti.

ALMOND BISCOTTI: Increase the vanilla to 2 teaspoons and replace the orange peel with 1 teaspoon almond flavoring.

LICORICE BISCOTTI: Increase the vanilla to 2 teaspoons and replace the orange peel with 1 teaspoon aniseed.

CHRISTMAS BISCOTTI: Replace the almonds with 1 1/2 cups chopped mixed candied fruit and 1/2 cup whole pine nuts.

CHOCOLATE-TOPPED BISCOTTI: For an added touch to any of the biscotti above, melt sweet chocolate and dip up to 1/4 inch of the rounded top of the cookie in the chocolate. You will have to roll this to make an even coat. Let dry on a slotted wire rack. (It takes practice to make the topping look professional, but it's well worth the trouble.)

LEBKUCHEN
(German Honey Cakes)

This spicy, moist rolled cookie is a great Christmas cookie; it can be made early in the season, before the rush of other baking. Lebkuchen should mellow in an airtight container for several days before being eaten.

1/2 cup molasses
1/2 cup honey
2/3 cup brown sugar
1 egg, beaten
1 tablespoon lemon juice
1 teaspoon grated lemon
rind
2 3/4 cups GF flour mix
1 teaspoon xanthan gum
1/2 teaspoon baking soda
1 teaspoon cinnamon
1 teaspoon cloves
1 teaspoon allspice
1 teaspoon nutmeg

1/2 cup candied fruits or
citron, diced fine
1/2 cup slivered almonds,
chopped
Whole almonds or candied
cherries, for decorating

Glaze

1 egg white, slightly beaten
1 teaspoon lemon juice
1 teaspoon grated lemon
rind
Dash salt
3/4 cup confectioner's sugar

Preheat oven to 350°.

In a small saucepan, bring molasses and honey to boil. Remove from heat and pour into a large mixing bowl. Let cool.

Stir in sugar, egg, lemon juice, and lemon rind.

In a separate bowl, blend the flour, xanthan gum, baking soda, cinnamon, cloves, allspice, and nutmeg, and add this to the molasses mixture, stirring until well blended. Stir in the candied fruits and almonds. Chill for several hours or overnight.

To shape cookies, work in small batches, keeping rest of the dough refrigerated. If dough is sticky, work in some rice flour. Roll out on a rice-floured board to 1/8 inch thick. Cut into 1 1/2-by-2-inch rectangles. Transfer to greased cookie sheets. Decorate with a single almond in the center or (as I prefer) with 2 or 3 thin slices of candied cherry on a slant down cookies, like the stripes on a barber pole.

Bake for 10 to 12 minutes, or until very lightly browned.

Glaze: Combine the egg white with the lemon juice, lemon rind, salt, and confectioner's sugar. Brush over hot cookies. Then transfer cookies to wax paper to cool.

For flavors to meld, store in an airtight container with a piece of apple or orange for several days. Remember to change fruit every few days so it does not become moldy. *Makes 5½ to 6 dozen cookies.*

MARY'S LEBKUCHEN BALLS: The tester who suggested these makes an entirely different (but good!) cookie from the same recipe. Eliminate the candied fruit and use nutmeats of your choice. Roll the dough into balls around each nut and bake. Do not decorate or glaze.

CHOCOLATE SURPRISE ROUNDS

If you're a peanut butter or chocolate fan, don't miss these chocolate cookies with a surprise layer of peanut butter filling baked in the middle. These take a bit of extra effort to make but are well worth the trouble. If desired, frost with a confectioner's sugar icing or decorate simply (as I do) with a lightning-shaped zigzag of the icing across the top of cookie.

Dough

1½ cups GF flour mix
¾ teaspoon xanthan gum
½ teaspoon salt
½ cup unsweetened cocoa
½ teaspoon baking soda
½ cup granulated sugar
½ cup brown sugar
½ cup (1 stick) butter or margarine
¼ cup creamy peanut butter

1 teaspoon vanilla
1 egg

Filling

¾ cup creamy peanut butter
¾ cup confectioner's sugar

Granulated sugar, for dipping

Preheat oven to 375°.

In a small bowl, combine the flour, xanthan gum, salt, cocoa, and baking soda. Blend well and set aside.

In a large mixing bowl, beat the sugars, butter, and peanut butter until light and fluffy. Add the vanilla and egg, beating well. Stir in the flour mixture until blended. Refrigerate while making filling.

In a small bowl, combine the peanut butter and confectioner's sugar. Blend well. Using your hands, form thirty 1-inch balls of the filling.

To make the cookies, shape about 1 tablespoonful of dough into a round, flat pattie. Place a filling ball in the center and ease the dough around it, covering completely. Place on an ungreased cookie sheet, spacing the balls about 2 inches apart. With the bottom of a glass dipped in sugar, flatten each ball to a little less than 1/4 inch thick. This will yield a 2 1/2- to 3-inch cookie when baked.

Bake for 7 to 9 minutes, or until set and slightly cracked. Remove immediately to cool before frosting (if desired). *Makes 30 cookies.*

CRESCENT CRISPS

A crisp cookie with a special crunch ingredient. These have a wonderful flavor and texture but are so "short" they aren't good travelers because they break easily.

1 cup (2 sticks) butter or margarine	1 1/2 cups rice flour
2/3 cup sugar	1/2 cup soy flour
1 teaspoon vanilla	1 1/2 cups crushed potato
1 egg	chips

Preheat oven to 350°.

In a large mixing bowl, beat the butter, sugar, and vanilla until fluffy. Beat in the egg.

Blend the rice flour, soy flour, and crushed potato chips. Stir into the egg-butter mix. The dough will be firm.

Pinch out enough dough to roll into a 1-inch ball; roll the ball to form a 2-inch-long piece with a slightly thickened center. Place on an ungreased cookie sheet and bend into a crescent. Repeat, leaving about 1 inch between cookies.

Bake for 16 to 18 minutes, or until lightly browned. Remove to cool; store in an airtight container. *Makes about 4 dozen crescents.*

PIES AND PASTRIES

PASTRY AND PIE CRUSTS

Donna Jo's Dream
  Pastry
Melt-in-the-Mouth Oil
  Crust
Mock Graham Cracker
  Crust
Ricotta Pastry
Absolutely Sinful Cereal
  Crust

REFRIGERATOR OR FREEZER PIES

Fresh Strawberry
  Pie
Eskimo Pie (or Ice
  Cream Bars)
Peanut Butter Pie with
  Chocolate Crust

BAKED PIES

Apple Pie Imperial
Fruit Cheesecake Pie
Caribbean Lime Pie
Lemon-Buttermilk Pie
Impossible German
  Chocolate Pie
Crustless Coconut Pie
Walnut-Cranberry Pie
Raspberry-Rhubarb Tart
  with Ricotta Crust

CRISP

Cranberry-Apple Crisp

PASTRIES

Danish Kringle
  Fresh Fruit Kringle
Fruit Danish
Bear Claws with Fig and
  Raisin Filling

Although fruit-filled pies seem acceptable for our diet, they usually have wheat-based crusts, so we have to pass them up when dining out. But we can make our own pastry.

I've given recipes for several crusts, including a new, tender pastry so good that your friends will never suspect it's gluten free. And there are other crusts, ranging from one made with our own Mock Graham Crackers to an Absolutely Sinful Cereal Crust. Also included are several pies that don't call for a crust at all.

Since fruit fillings can be made gluten free, I've included only a few excitingly different ones for your pies. If you use your old fruit-pie recipe, be sure to thicken it with cornstarch, tapioca, or rice flour. For even easier fillings, you can find many GF puddings and pie fillings on the market, but, since companies do change formulas, always check the ingredients list before using these.

This section also contains some delicious breakfast pastries you probably thought you'd never eat again: the Danish breakfast roll, a fruit-filled kringle, and bear claws.

If a recipe calls for my GF flour mix, here is the formula:

2 parts white rice flour
2/3 part potato starch flour
1/3 part tapioca flour

PASTRY AND PIE CRUSTS

DONNA JO'S DREAM PASTRY

Finally, a successful pie crust! In my first book, I had to admit that my Tender Vinegar Pastry was hard to cut. This one, with its variety of flours, is successful every time and can be cut either hot or cold. For perfect results, follow the directions carefully and chill the dough one hour or more before rolling.

$^1/_2$ cup tapioca flour
$^1/_2$ cup cornstarch
$^1/_4$ cup potato starch flour
1 cup sweet rice flour
1 rounded teaspoon
  xanthan gum
$^1/_2$ teaspoon salt
Dash sugar (optional)

$^1/_2$ cup (1 stick) margarine
$^1/_2$ cup Butter Flavor
  Crisco
1 egg, cold
1 tablespoon GF vinegar
4 tablespoons ice water
Sweet rice flour, for rolling

Blend together the flours, xanthan gum, salt, and sugar. Cut in the margarine and Crisco in small dabs until you have shortening the size of lima beans (not cornmeal).

Beat the egg using a fork; add the vinegar and ice water. Stir into the flour mixture, forming a ball. You may knead this a bit, since rice flour crusts can stand handling. Refrigerate the dough for an hour or more to chill.

Divide dough and roll out on a sweet rice–floured board (or on floured plastic wrap, for easier handling). Place in a pie tin. If using plastic wrap, remove it to the pie tin and invert the dough into the pan. Shape before removing the plastic. Bake as directed for the filling used.

For a baked crust, prick the pastry with a fork on sides and bottom. Bake the crust in a preheated 450° oven for 10 to 12 minutes, or until slightly browned. Cool before filling. *Makes enough pastry for a 2-crust 9″ pie plus 1 pie shell.*

MELT-IN-THE-MOUTH
OIL CRUST

This easy pat-into-the-pan crust is so simple to make, it may become your favorite for single-crust pies. This is not flaky but does cut well and is guaranteed to melt in your mouth (with no gritty aftertaste).

1 cup sweet rice flour	1¹/₄ teaspoons salt
¹/₂ cup tapioca flour	²/₃ cup vegetable oil
¹/₂ cup cornstarch	3 tablespoons cold milk or
1 teaspoon xanthan gum	nondairy liquid
1¹/₂ teaspoons sugar	(NutQuik, great!)
(optional)	

In a medium bowl, mix together flours, xanthan gum, sugar (if used), and salt.

Pour the oil into a measuring cup and whip in the milk with a fork until the two are blended. Pour into the flour mixture and blend lightly until well moistened. (The dough will not form a ball.)

Pat the mixture into a 9″ or 10″ oiled pie tin. Form a medium thick crust, shaping the edges and fluting the top, if desired.

If the pie is to be filled and then baked, pour the filling in gently and bake as directed for the filling used.

For a baked crust, bake the crust in a preheated 425° oven for about 15 minutes, or until golden. Cool before filling. *Makes one 9″ or 10″ pie shell.*

MOCK GRAHAM
CRACKER CRUST

If a recipe calls for a graham cracker crust, this mock version will fool anyone. It is easy to make if you already have the Mock Graham Crackers. For added taste, add ground almonds.

> 1¹/₂ cups finely crushed Mock Graham Crackers (page 84)
> 4 tablespoons (¹/₂ stick) butter or margarine, melted
> ¹/₄ cup finely ground almonds (optional)

Place the cracker crumbs in a plastic bag. Add the butter and almonds (if used) and shake together. Pat the mixture into and up the sides of a 9″ pie tin. Bake as directed for the filling used.

If the filling is already cooked, bake the crust in a preheated 375° oven for 6 to 8 minutes. Check after 6 minutes to prevent the crust from browning too much. Cool before filling. *Makes one 9″ pie shell.*

RICOTTA PASTRY

A rich, flaky pastry crust especially good with fruit fillings. This makes a large recipe and can be halved for a single pie. Or, do as I do, and make a pie from half and use the other half in one of the kringles (pages 162–63).

> 1¹/₂ cups white rice flour
> ¹/₂ cup tapioca flour
> 1 teaspoon baking powder
> 1 teaspoon xanthan gum
> 1 cup (2 sticks) margarine,
>   melted
>
> ¹/₂ cup ricotta cheese
> ¹/₂ cup sour cream
>   (no substitute)

In a medium mixing bowl, sift together the flours, baking powder, and xanthan gum. Stir in the margarine and add the ricotta cheese and sour cream. The mixture will look more like cooked cereal than pastry dough. Chill for at least 2 hours, or until the dough is firm and easy to handle.

Roll out the dough on rice-floured plastic for easy handling. I usually cover it with a second piece of plastic wrap so the dough doesn't stick to the rolling pin. To place in the pie tin, remove the top plastic and use the second to invert the dough into the pan. Shape before removing the plastic. Bake as directed for the filling used.

For a baked crust, prick the pastry with a fork on sides and bottom. Bake in a preheated 400° oven for about 25 minutes, or until the crust is flaky and lightly browned. Cool before filling. *Makes enough pastry for a 2-crust pie plus 1 extra crust or kringle.*

ABSOLUTELY SINFUL CEREAL CRUST

This crust was named by the first person who tasted it—and she wasn't even a celiac. Use it for any of your open-faced pies, whether they be fruit, pumpkin, or custard cream, but be prepared to cut the pieces smaller than usual, for this is a rich crust! Try this also for cheesecake. If macaroon coconut (a fine grind) is not available in your local health food store, use flaked or shredded coconut and chop it finer in a food processor.

3 tablespoons butter or margarine, melted	1 cup GF cornflakes, crushed
2/3 cup brown sugar	2/3 cup macaroon coconut
1 cup Kenmai Rice Bran, crushed	2/3 cup walnuts, ground fine

Stir together all the ingredients. Line a deep 9″ greased pie tin with the mix, patting well up the sides. Or pat into a 10″ springform pan for cheesecake. Bake as directed for the filling used.

If the filling is already cooked, bake in a preheated 375° oven for 6 minutes, or until the crust is slightly browned. Cool before filling. *Makes 1 deep 9″ pie crust or a 10″ cheesecake crust.*

REFRIGERATOR OR FREEZER PIES

FRESH STRAWBERRY PIE

A wonderful treat during strawberry season. This pie uses one baked pie shell and needs to chill two hours in the refrigerator before serving. You can purchase a glaze that might be gluten free, but it will not have the fresh flavor of this easy, home-cooked version.

One 8-inch baked pie
  shell
1 quart fresh
  strawberries

Glaze

1/2 cup sugar
1/2 teaspoon salt
1/2 cup water

1 1/2 tablespoons cornstarch
1 tablespoon lemon juice

Filling

One 8-ounce package
  cream cheese, softened
2 tablespoons milk or
  nondairy liquid
3 tablespoons sugar

Prepare the crust.

Wash and hull the berries. Slice all but 5 of them.

Glaze: In a small saucepan, put 1 cup of the sliced berries, 1/2 cup sugar, salt, and 1/4 cup of the water. Bring to a boil and cook for 3 minutes. Remove from heat. Mix the cornstarch and the remaining 1/4 cup cold water. Stir into the berry mixture and return to heat, stirring until thick and clear, about 2 minutes. Remove from heat, add lemon juice, and let cool.

Filling: Beat the cream cheese with the milk and sugar. Spread in the bottom of the pie shell. Cover with a third of the glaze. Top with the remaining sliced berries. Cut the 5 whole berries in half and form a circle in the center of the fruit with tips facing out. Top with the remaining glaze. Chill for at least 2 hours (overnight is fine). *Makes 6 servings.*

ESKIMO PIE
(or Ice Cream Bars)

Make this easy nut-packed, crunchy crust with a frozen filling into a pie, or freeze into ice cream–like bars.

1/2 cup butter or margarine, melted	1 cup flaked coconut
1 cup brown sugar	1 cup walnuts, chopped fine
1 1/2 cups Kenmai Rice Bran, crushed	1 quart GF vanilla ice cream, frozen yogurt, or nondairy substitute
1 1/2 cups GF cornflakes, crushed	

Combine the butter, sugar, rice bran, cornflakes, coconut, and nuts. Pat two-thirds of the mixture, in either a deep 9″ pie tin or a 9″ × 13″ baking pan. Fill with the ice cream, yogurt, or nondairy substitute. Cover with the remaining cereal mixture, pressing lightly into the filling. Freeze for several hours or overnight.

This is a rich dessert, so you may wish to cut the pie into 8 to 12 wedges and the flat pan into 9 to 12 bars. You may wrap the bars separately and freeze for eating singly.

PEANUT BUTTER PIE WITH CHOCOLATE CRUST

This rich, no-bake pie with an easy-to-make cereal crust can serve up to ten guests. If you don't have macaroon coconut, substitute flaked or shredded coconut and chop it finer in a food processor. The pie needs at least four hours in the refrigerator before serving.

Crust

1¹/₂ cups GF cereal, crushed
¹/₃ cup macaroon coconut
¹/₃ cup brown sugar
2 tablespoons cocoa
4 tablespoons (¹/₂ stick) butter or margarine, melted

Filling

¹/₂ cup chunk-style peanut butter

¹/₂ cup sugar
One 8-ounce package cream cheese, room temperature
2 cups nondairy whipped topping or 1 cup whipping, cream, whipped, plus 2 tablespoons sugar

Preheat oven to 375°.

Make the crust by combining the cereal, coconut, sugar, and cocoa in a bowl or plastic bag. Mix in the butter. Pat the mixture into a deep 9″ or 10″ pie tin. Bake for 6 to 8 minutes, or until crust is slightly browned. Cool before filling.

To make the filling, beat together the peanut butter, sugar, and cream cheese until blended. Fold in the whipped topping. Pour into the cooled pie crust and refrigerate for at least 4 hours before serving. *Makes 8 to 10 servings.*

BAKED PIES

APPLE PIE IMPERIAL

Wonderful! An easy batter topping with streusel makes this an extra-special pie, and there's no crust to roll. The almond flavor is enhanced by the use of NutQuik or ground almonds.

Filling

4 or 5 apples, pared and
    sliced (approximately
    5 cups)
1 teaspoon cinnamon
1/4 teaspoon nutmeg
1 cup sugar

Batter

1/2 cup sweet rice flour
1/4 cup cornstarch
2 teaspoons baking
    powder
1/2 teaspoon salt

3 tablespoons NutQuik
    granules or 3
    tablespoons ground
    almonds
1/2 cup water
2 eggs
2 tablespoons margarine or
    butter, melted

Streusel Topping

1/2 cup brown sugar
4 tablespoons (1/2 stick)
    margarine or butter
1/2 cup chopped almonds

Preheat oven to 325°.

Tumble the apples with the cinnamon, nutmeg, and sugar. Place evenly in a deep, buttered 9″ pie tin.

In a small bowl, blend together the flour, cornstarch, baking powder, and salt. With a blender, mix the NutQuik and the water.

In a medium bowl, beat the eggs, margarine, and water mixture. Add the flour mixture and beat until smooth. Pour the batter over the apples.

In a small bowl, blend together the sugar, margarine, and nuts until they are crumbly. Sprinkle this streusel over the batter. Bake the pie for approximately 45 minutes, or until the apples are cooked. This is a rich dessert providing 8 to 10 servings.

FRUIT CHEESECAKE PIE

Fresh fruit in season plus a cheesecake custard topping make this a rich, mouth-watering dessert for a crowd. Change the flavor with your choice of fruits—spring rhubarb, winter apples, local cherries, or exotic pineapple. You should refrigerate the pie at least two hours or longer before serving.

Mock Graham Cracker Crust, (page 148) or cereal crust (page 149)

Fruit Layer

3 cups fresh fruit (cherries, rhubarb, pineapple, etc.)
1 tablespoon water
2/3 cup sugar
2 tablespoons cornstarch
1 teaspoon flavored gelatin, for color

Cheesecake Topping

Two 3-ounce packages cream cheese, softened
2 eggs
1 tablespoon lemon juice
6 tablespoons sugar
1 cup sour cream or nondairy substitute

Preheat oven to 350°.

Prepare the crust (reserving 2 tablespoons of the mixture). Do not bake.

Prepare the fruit by cutting the rhubarb into 1/2-inch slices, pitting the cherries or peeling, coring, and cutting the pineapple into small (1/2 inch or less) tidbits.

In a 2-quart saucepan, mix together the selected fruit, the water, sugar, and cornstarch. (Eliminate the water if the fruit is *very* juicy.) Cook, stirring often over medium heat, until the mixture comes to a full boil. Remove from heat and add the gelatin (raspberry for rhubarb, cherry for cherry, and lemon for apple and pineapple). Pour the fruit mixture into the prepared crust.

With a mixer, blend together the cream cheese, eggs, lemon juice, sugar, and sour cream. Pour over the fruit filling. Top with a sprinkling of the reserved crumb mix.

Bake for 25 to 30 minutes, or until the center appears set when shaken gently.

Cool and then refrigerate from 2 to 24 hours before serving. *Makes 10 to 12 servings.*

CARIBBEAN LIME PIE

A tasty, tangy lime taste, very different from the sweet, milk-filled traditional Key lime pie. You can find the genuine Key lime juice at some larger supermarkets. I prefer the graham cracker crust, but a cereal crust (see page 149) also tastes good. This needs to chill in the refrigerator two hours before serving.

1 Mock Graham Cracker
   Crust (page 148), baked
   10 minutes
5 eggs, separated
1¹/₄ cups sugar
²/₃ cup Key lime juice

1 tablespoon grated lime
   peel or lemon peel
Salt to taste
Whipped cream or
   nondairy substitute,
   for topping

Preheat oven to 350°.

Prepare the crust.

In the top of a double boiler, beat the egg yolks until thick. Gradually beat in 1 cup of the sugar. Beat until pale yellow. Add the lime juice and rind. Place over a pan of hot water and cook until thick enough to coat a spoon, about 8 minutes. Remove from water and cool.

Add a pinch of salt to the egg whites and beat until they form soft peaks. Gradually beat in the last ¹/₄ cup of sugar. Beat until stiff. Blend a third of the beaten whites into the cooked mixture; fold in the remaining whites.

Pour the filling into the prepared crust and bake for 15 minutes. The pie will set more as it cools. Cool and refrigerate for at least 2 hours before serving. Top with whipped cream or nondairy topping. *Makes one 9" pie or 6 servings.*

LEMON-BUTTERMILK PIE

A delicious updated version of an old Scandinavian recipe, this uses one unbaked pie shell. It pairs perfectly with Donna Jo's Dream Pastry (page 146), or the Melt-in-the-Mouth Oil Crust (page 147). I use reconstituted powdered buttermilk and have excellent results.

1 unbaked pie shell	3 tablespoons butter or
3 eggs, separated	margarine, melted
3/4 cup sugar, divided	1 1/2 cups buttermilk
2 tablespoons sweet rice	3 tablespoons lemon juice
flour	1 tablespoon fresh grated
1/4 teaspoon salt	lemon peel

Preheat oven to 350°.

Prepare the pie crust in deep 9″ pie tin.

In a medium mixing bowl, beat the egg whites until foamy. Add 1/4 cup of the sugar and beat until soft peaks form. Set aside.

In another mixing bowl, beat together the egg yolks, the remaining 1/2 cup sugar, the rice flour, salt, and butter. Beat in the buttermilk, lemon juice, and grated peel.

Gently fold in the egg white mixture and pour the filling into the prepared pie crust. Bake for 25 to 30 minutes, or until a knife inserted in the center comes out clean and the pie is slightly toasted looking on top. Cool before serving. *Makes 6 servings.*

IMPOSSIBLE GERMAN
CHOCOLATE PIE

A chocoholic's dream filled with coconut and pecans. And there is no crust to make! The recipe came from a tester who was trying to make an easy, lactose-free company dessert. She was so successful that a dozen were served to rave reviews on shipboard at the first Celiac Experience.

1¹/₂ cup nondairy liquid (Mocha Mix, Coffee Rich, Farm Rich, or other; see Note)	¹/₂ teaspoon salt
	¹/₄ teaspoon vanilla
	¹/₄ cup rice flour
	3 eggs
One 4-ounce bar German sweet chocolate, melted	²/₃ cup sugar
	¹/₂ cup chopped pecans
¹/₄ cup (¹/₂ stick) margarine, softened	1 cup shredded coconut

Preheat oven to 350°.

In a blender or food processor, place all ingredients except the nuts and coconut. Blend for 3 minutes. Stir in the pecans and coconut.

Pour into a deep, greased 9″ pie tin and bake for 30 to 35 minutes, or until set. Chill before serving. *Makes 8 servings.*

NOTE: For those intolerant or allergic to soy, NutQuik liquid may be substituted.

CRUSTLESS COCONUT PIE

An easy, delicious coconut dessert from the Philippines.

1 cup sugar	1¹/₂ cups rich milk or
1 cup flaked coconut	nondairy liquid
¹/₂ cup GF flour mix	¹/₂ cup sour cream or
³/₄ teaspoon baking	nondairy substitute
powder	2 tablespoons butter or
¹/₄ teaspoon salt	margarine, melted
Dash nutmeg	1 teaspoon vanilla
4 eggs, beaten	

Preheat oven to 325°.

In a medium bowl, blend together the sugar, coconut, flour, baking powder, salt, and nutmeg. Set aside.

In a large bowl, beat the eggs. Add the milk, sour cream, butter, and vanilla. Beat slightly until smooth. Stir in the dry ingredients and pour into a deep 9″ buttered pie tin. Bake for 55 to 60 minutes, or until tester inserted in center comes out clean. *Makes 8 servings.*

WALNUT-CRANBERRY PIE

A rich nut pie with cranberries to provide contrast and a jewel-dotted look to the filling. This calls for one deep 9" unbaked pastry or cereal crust.

1 unbaked pie shell
3 eggs
²/₃ cup dark corn syrup
³/₄ cup dark brown sugar, packed
6 tablespoons (³/₄ stick) butter or margarine, melted

1 teaspoon brandy or GF vanilla flavoring
1¹/₄ cups cranberries, fresh or frozen
1¹/₂ cups walnuts, chopped coarsely
Whipped cream topping (optional)

Preheat oven to 350°.

In a large mixing bowl, beat the eggs slightly. Add the corn syrup, sugar, butter, and brandy, and mix well. Fold in the cranberries and nuts. Pour into the prepared pie crust.

Bake for 50 to 55 minutes, or until a knife inserted in the center comes out clean. Cool before serving. Top with whipped cream (if desired). *Makes 6 to 8 servings.*

RASPBERRY-RHUBARB TART
WITH RICOTTA CRUST

A perfect foil for the winter blahs, the bright red filling will bring spring into your kitchen; the taste will bring delight. Use the extra trimmings from the crust for top decorations.

3 to 4 cups fresh or frozen rhubarb, in $1/2$-inch slices
One 10-ounce package frozen raspberries in syrup
1 cup sugar, or to taste

1 tablespoon lemon juice
3 tablespoons cornstarch
1 teaspoon apple pie spice
$1/2$ recipe Ricotta Pastry (page 148)
1 tablespoon butter or margarine, melted

In a large mixing bowl, tumble the rhubarb, raspberries, sugar, lemon juice, cornstarch, and apple pie spice. Let set for about 30 minutes.

Preheat oven to 400°.

Prepare the crust by rolling out on rice-floured pastry cloth or plastic. Place in 9″ pie tin or tart pan. Shape and trim. Reroll the trimmings and cut with a cookie cutter into 5 shapes of your choice (hearts for Valentine's Day, circles, or half-moons, for example). Put the cut dough aside for top decorations.

To the fruit mixture add the butter and pour the mixture into the shell. Top with the crust decorations. Bake for 45 to 55 minutes, or until the crust is slightly browned and the filling is bubbly. Cool before serving. *Makes 6 servings.*

CRISP

CRANBERRY-APPLE CRISP

Serve this flavorful easy-to-make crisp to any guests and they'll never suspect it's gluten free.

Filling

4 to 5 cups peeled, cored, and sliced cooking apples
1 cup fresh or frozen cranberries
2/3 cup sugar
2 teaspoons cinnamon
1 teaspoon allspice
2 tablespoons brandy

Topping

1 cup sliced almonds, crushed
2/3 cup dark brown sugar
1/3 cup white rice flour
1/4 cup (1/2 stick) butter, melted
Whipped cream, frozen yogurt, or ice cream, for topping (optional)

Preheat oven to 350°.

Tumble together the apples, cranberries, sugar, cinnamon, and allspice. Pour into an 8″ square glass baking dish with 2″ sides. Microwave on high for 4 to 5 minutes, stirring several times. Remove and stir in the brandy.

For topping, blend together the almonds, sugar, flour, and butter. Crumble this mixture over the top of the fruit. Bake for 25 to 30 minutes, or until the top is slightly brown and the juice oozes up around the edges. Remove and let set 10 minutes to finish cooking.

Serve hot or cold in glass dessert dishes topped, if desired, with the whipped cream or ice cream. *Makes 6 to 8 servings.*

PASTRIES

DANISH KRINGLE

This easy-to-make, rich pastry can take many different fillings to become a coffee-break snack, a dinner dessert, or a sweet for evening munching.

Pastry
1¹/₂ cups white rice
 flour
¹/₂ cup tapioca flour
1 teaspoon baking powder
1 teaspoon xanthan gum
1 cup (2 sticks) margarine,
 melted
¹/₂ cup ricotta cheese

¹/₂ cup sour cream
 (no substitute)

Filling
1 can of any GF pie filling

Topping
¹/₂ cup confectioner's sugar
1 to 1¹/₂ tablespoons milk

In a medium mixing bowl, sift together the flours, baking powder, and xanthan gum. Stir in the margarine; add the ricotta cheese and sour cream. This will look more like cooked cereal than pastry dough. Chill for at least 2 hours, or until the dough becomes firm and easy to handle.

Preheat oven to 400°.

Divide dough in half and roll out the sections, one at a time, on rice-floured plastic to a rectangle approximately 10 by 16 inches. Spoon half the can of filling down the center of the long measurement. Lifting with the plastic, fold one side (one-third) of the dough over the filling, then fold the other side. Pinch both ends into rounded points and seal them by pressing. Using the plastic to lift, turn the kringle over onto one side of an ungreased cookie sheet. Repeat with the second half of the dough. Slash through the tops in diagonal slits about every 1¹/₂ to 2 inches and bake for 35 to 40 minutes, or until browned and flaky.

Mix the confectioner's sugar and milk. While the pastry is still hot, drizzle on the topping. Serve either hot or cold. (These may be frozen to serve later.) *Each kringle serves 6.*

FRESH FRUIT KRINGLE: For the filling, use 3½ cups of any peeled and sliced fresh fruit (apricot or prune are traditional, but I have used peaches, apples, cherries, and pineapple). Mix the fruit with ⅓ cup of sugar (or to taste) plus 1 tablespoon cornstarch. Cook 5 to 6 minutes on high in a microwave, stirring once or twice.

FRUIT DANISH

The sweet, fruited breakfast roll we've been hungering for when others are enjoying the store-bought ones. These are easy to make, with no kneading and only one rising. If you use rapid-rise yeast, the rolls can be mixed, raised, and baked in less than 45 minutes. Lemon curd is available in most large markets.

1½ cups GF flour mix	1 egg plus 1 egg yolk,
1½ teaspoons baking	room temperature
powder	¾ cup jam (raspberry,
1 teaspoon xanthan gum	pineapple, apricot) or
½ teaspoon salt	lemon curd
3 tablespoons sugar	
1 cup lukewarm water	*Icing*
1 tablespoon dry yeast	½ cup confectioner's sugar
granules	1 tablespoon butter
3 tablespoons margarine or	1 tablespoon milk (or to
butter, melted	desired consistency)

In a small bowl, mix together the flour, baking powder, xanthan gum, and salt. Set aside.

Mix 1 teaspoon of the sugar into the water, then stir in the yeast. Set aside until it foams slightly.

In a large mixing bowl, blend together with a hand mixer at low speed the remaining sugar, margarine, eggs, and yeast mixture. Beat in half the flour mixture. Stir in the rest of the flour and beat with a spoon until the batter is smooth.

Spoon 6 flat rounds of batter onto a greased cookie tin. Swirl a circular depression in each round of dough and fill with approximately 2 tablespoons of the desired filling. Cover and let rise in a warm place until the batter doubles, 40 to 45 minutes for regular yeast, 20 minutes for rapid rise. Preheat oven to 375°.

Bake for 20 to 23 minutes, or until slightly browned. Do not overbake or the filling will be dry.

To make the icing, combine all ingredients. Drizzle onto the danishes while they are still hot.

Makes 6 servings.

BEAR CLAWS WITH FIG
AND RAISIN FILLING

A rich, filled pastry for breakfast, brunch, or just snacking, the bear claw is good hot or cold, iced or plain. Make up the crust and refrigerate it while you cook the filling.

1 recipe Ricotta Pastry
(page 148)

Filling

1/2 cup dried figs, chopped
fine
1/2 cup raisins
1 cup water
3 tablespoons butter or
margarine

1/2 cup brown sugar
1 teaspoon vanilla
1/2 teaspoon dried orange
peel
1/2 cup chopped walnuts

Icing (optional)

Confectioner's sugar
Milk

Mix the crust ingredients, form ball, and refrigerate.

Filling: In a small saucepan, combine the figs, raisins, and water. Bring to a boil. Lower heat to a simmer and cook for 15 minutes.

Remove from heat and beat in the butter, sugar, vanilla, and orange peel. Then add the nuts.

Preheat oven to 400°.

To shape the pastries, divide the crust ball in half and roll out, a section at a time, on rice-floured plastic to a rectangle approximately 10 by 16 inches. Place half the filling in 5 separate sections down the center of the long measurement. Lifting the plastic, fold one side, one-third, of the dough over the filling, then repeat with the other side. Seal both ends and pinch the dough between the filled sections. Cut apart at the pinched areas.

Using a spatula, place the pieces on ungreased cookie sheets, reversing the dough so the smooth side is up. Slash twice, diagonally, across each pastry. Repeat with the second half of the dough and bake for 35 to 40 minutes, or until lightly browned.

While still hot, drizzle on a thin icing of confectioner's sugar and milk, if desired. *Makes 10 bear claws.*

DESSERTS

BAKED AND SHAPED DESSERTS

Pam's Pavlova
Swedish Apple Torte
Linzertorte
Almond-Lace Dessert Cups

NO-BAKE DESSERTS

Four-Layer Dessert
Pistachio Bars
Down-Under Trifle

PUDDINGS

Creamy Rice Pudding
Spicy Bread Pudding
Apple Pudding
    Rum-flavored Whipped
    Cream
Rhubarb Fool

As my family gathered around the dinner table when I was a child, my brothers never asked, "What's for dinner?" It was always, "What's for dessert?" They wondered if they should save room for a special treat or eat their fill of the meat and potatoes and, if they had a corner empty, finish on the usual home-canned fruit.

I wondered, too, because if dessert was to be a cake, bread pudding, or even a fruit dumpling, I'd skip it. Even then, more than forty years before I'd heard of celiac sprue, for me, eating the cake, pudding, or dumpling would cause a sleepless night. My parents figured I was sensitive to sugar. Now I realize I already showed symptoms of gluten intolerance and avoided foods that brought on reactions.

I was envious of my brothers and my sister. Now they can envy me. Other chapters in the book have recipes for out-of-this-world cakes and wonderful cookies; in this chapter I've gathered a wide variety of interesting sweets and, if they weren't already gluten free, have altered them to our diet.

For that little touch of something sweet to end the meal, there are puddings and fruits with custard sauce. For a special occasion, there are some "I-can't-believe-this-is-gluten-free" treats like Linzertorte, Pam's Pavlova, and Pistachio Bars so rich you must tell your guests ahead of time to save room for dessert.

BAKED AND SHAPED DESSERTS

PAM'S PAVLOVA

New Zealand's national dessert was first created by an inspired chef for the ballerina Pavlova's visit to that country. Now, according to my hostess in Auckland, there are as many recipes for the dessert as there are cooks in the country. She shared her recipe with me. The long beating is her secret. The center should be soft, the outside a crusty meringue. She says there's never a failure, for however it turns out, that is the way it should be.

4 egg whites, room
   temperature
1¹/₂ cups fine sugar
1 teaspoon cornstarch
1 teaspoon vinegar
1 teaspoon vanilla

Topping
3 kiwifruit
1 cup whipping cream plus
   3 tablespoons sugar, or
   2 cups nondairy
   whipped topping
¹/₂ cup strawberries or
   other fresh fruit

Preheat oven to 250° to 275°.

In a large mixing bowl (metal or glass), beat the egg whites until soft peaks form. Add half the sugar and beat for 10 minutes. Fold in the cornstarch, vinegar, vanilla, and remaining sugar. Pile on an oven tray that has been covered with aluminum foil and shape as desired, either in a mound or cake shape. Bake for 1¹/₂ hours, or until crusty outside and lightly browned. Remove and cool.

Peel and slice the kiwifruit and whip the cream. Frost the cake with the cream and arrange the kiwifruit and strawberries or other fruit on top. Strawberries and raspberries should be tumbled in sugar before being added to the Pavlova; peaches, bananas, and other non-acidic fruits are better added just before serving. Cut in wedges to serve. *Makes 8 generous servings.*

SWEDISH APPLE TORTE

This cross between a cake and pie makes a refreshingly different dessert that is rich tasting and moist, and can be served either hot or cold. For a different flavor, try using almonds, macadamia, or cashews rather than the walnuts.

1¹/₂ cups finely chopped
  apple (2 apples)
¹/₂ teaspoon cinnamon
¹/₄ teaspoon cloves
1 tablespoon butter or
  margarine, melted
1 tablespoon lemon juice
²/₃ cup sugar
¹/₂ cup rice flour
1 teaspoon baking powder

¹/₄ teaspoon salt
1 egg, beaten
¹/₃ cup sour cream or
  nondairy substitute
¹/₂ cup chopped walnuts or
  pecans
Whipped cream or
  nondairy whipped
  topping

Preheat oven to 350°.

Place the apple, cinnamon, cloves, butter, and lemon juice in a glass dish and microwave on high for 5 minutes, stirring once.

Blend together the sugar, flour, baking powder, and salt. Stir into the partially cooked apples.

Mix the egg with sour cream, and add along with the nuts to the batter. Pour into a greased pie tin and bake for 30 minutes, or until the top springs back when touched lightly.

Cut in wedges to serve either hot or cold topped with whipped cream. *Makes 6 servings.*

LINZERTORTE

The classic Austrian favorite adapts well to our flours but is still rich, so cut the pieces small. This easy version doesn't require rolling the dough. Although the traditional linzertorte is made with raspberry filling, you can substitute peach or apricot preserves.

3 eggs, room temperature
$1/2$ cup cornstarch
$1/2$ cup sweet rice flour
$1/4$ cup potato starch flour
$1/2$ teaspoon xanthan gum
$1/2$ teaspoon salt
1 teaspoon dried lemon peel
$1/2$ cup butter or margarine

$1/2$ cup granulated sugar
$1^1/2$ cups ground almonds, divided
$1/3$ teaspoon cream of tartar
1 cup confectioner's sugar, sifted
$1/2$ cup raspberry preserves

Preheat oven to 350°.

Separate the eggs, placing the whites in a medium bowl. Set aside.

In a smaller bowl, blend together the cornstarch, flours, xanthan gum, salt, and lemon peel.

In a medium bowl, beat the butter until softened. Add half the flour mixture and the granulated sugar and egg yolks. Beat on medium speed until thoroughly combined. Stir in the remaining flour and $1/2$ cup of the ground almonds. Press this crust into the bottom and 1 inch up the sides of a 9″ springform pan and bake for 15 minutes.

Meanwhile, add the cream of tartar to the egg whites and, using clean beaters, beat on medium speed until soft peaks form. Gradually add the confectioner's sugar and beat until stiff peaks form. Fold in the remaining 1 cup almonds.

Spread the raspberry preserves over the hot baked crust; top with the meringue. Return to the oven and bake for about 20 minutes longer, or until the top is golden brown. Cool. Cut in small wedges to serve. *Makes 12 to 16 servings.*

ALMOND-LACE DESSERT CUPS

These delicate and delicious made-to-eat dishes for ice cream, frozen yogurt, or fruit are a bit tricky to make, but will be well worth the time when you hear your guests rave. These can be made ahead and stored airtight for several days.

1/4 cup (1/2 stick) margarine or butter, melted	1 large egg
1/2 cup dark brown sugar, packed	1/4 cup finely ground almonds
	1 tablespoon white rice flour

Preheat oven to 300°.

Cut foil or cooking parchment into eight 6-inch squares and grease one side. Place, greased side up, 4 to a sheet, on 2 ungreased baking sheets.

In a medium bowl, beat together the butter, sugar, egg, nuts, and flour.

Divide batter among the 8 prepared squares and smooth each to about a 4-inch circle, which will spread during baking to about a 5-inch circle. Bake, a pan at a time, for about 15 minutes, or until the cookies are darkened slightly at the edges.

Let cool about 1 minute, then, while cookies are still flexible, peel off the foil or paper and immediately drape the cookie over the "cups" of an upside-down muffin tin. If the cookies are too stiff to drape well, return the tin to the oven for a few seconds to let them soften.

The cups can be stored in an airtight container for up to 3 days. *Makes 8 dessert cups.*

NO-BAKE DESSERTS

FOUR-LAYER DESSERT

This deliciously rich dessert is easy to make ahead for your next party. The only thing that requires baking is the simple crust.

Crust

4 tablespoons margarine, melted

1 cup crushed GF cereal or GF cookie crumbs

1 cup chopped walnuts, divided

Filling

One 8-ounce package cream cheese, softened

1 cup confectioner's sugar

One 8-ounce carton nondairy whipped topping

One 6-ounce package instant GF chocolate pudding (see Note)

2 cups milk

Preheat oven to 375°.

Crust: Add the margarine to the crushed cereal. Stir in 1/2 cup of the nuts. Spread the mixture in an ungreased 9″ × 13″ baking dish and bake for about 13 minutes, or until lightly browned. Be careful not to overcook. Cool.

Second layer: Combine the cream cheese, sugar, and 1 cup of the whipped topping. Spread over the cooled crust.

Third layer: Combine the pudding and milk. Beat until thick. Pour the mixture over the cream cheese layer.

Topping: Cover with the remaining whipped topping and sprinkle on the remaining 1/2 cup nuts. Refrigerate for at least 2 hours before serving. *Makes 10 to 12 servings.*

NOTE: Try this with butterscotch pudding for a caramel flavor.

PISTACHIO BARS

A rich-looking layered refrigerator dessert that can be made ahead for your next dinner party. Or take it to a potluck, for this feeds a large crowd. Don't be fooled by the layers; this is easy to make. If you don't have sweet rice flour, substitute GF cookie crumbs or crushed GF cereal.

First Layer

1 cup sweet rice flour
1/2 cup butter or margarine
2 tablespoons sugar
1/4 cup chopped walnuts

Second Layer

One 8-ounce package
   cream cheese, softened
1 cup plain yogurt
2/3 cup confectioner's sugar

Third Layer

Two 3.75-ounce packages
   GF instant pistachio
   pudding mix
2 1/2 cups cold milk (no
   substitute)

Fourth Layer

1 1/2 cups nondairy
   whipped topping
1/4 cup chopped walnuts

Preheat oven to 350°.

First layer: Mix together the ingredients and pat into a 9″ × 13″ pan. Bake for 10 to 15 minutes and let cool a few minutes.

Second layer: Soften and blend the cream cheese with the yogurt and confectioner's sugar. Spread over the first layer.

Third layer: With a hand mixer at medium speed, beat together the pudding mix and cold milk until the pudding is thick. Spread over the second layer.

Fourth layer: Top with the whipped topping and sprinkle with the remaining nuts.

Refrigerate at least 4 hours before serving (overnight is even better). *Makes 12 servings.*

DOWN-UNDER TRIFLE

A light, tangy trifle that can be made a day ahead instead of being put together at the last minute. A new twist to the old English dessert is added with the use of New Zealand kiwis, and since this turns out such a beautiful molded dessert, any topping is optional.

1 Sponge Roll (page 113; see Note)
1 envelope unflavored gelatin
1/2 cup cold water
3/4 cup lemon juice
1 1/4 cups sugar, divided
6 eggs, separated
2 tablespoons grated lemon rind
3 ripe kiwifruit, peeled and sliced
1 cup whipping cream or 4 ounces (1/2 carton) nondairy whipped topping

Topping (optional)
1 cup whipping cream or 4 ounces (1/2 carton) nondairy whipped topping
2 tablespoons rum
2 tablespoons sugar
1 pint strawberries, sliced and sugared

Using half the sponge roll, cut two 2 1/2-inch strips from the end. Cut these into 1/2-inch "fingers." Tear the remaining sponge roll into small (walnut-sized) pieces and place in a large mixing bowl.

Sprinkle gelatin over water in a small bowl.

In the top of a double boiler, mix the lemon juice with 1/2 cup of the sugar, egg yolks, and lemon rind. Stir and cook over hot water until thick, 7 to 8 minutes. Remove from heat and stir in the gelatin mixture. Set aside to cool.

Prepare a 10-inch (3-inch-high) springform pan by lining the bottom with the kiwi slices and standing the ladyfinger pieces of cake evenly around the sides.

Beat the egg whites until foamy. Slowly add the remaining 3/4 cup sugar, beating constantly, until the mixture is stiff. Fold in the cooled yolk mixture.

Whip the cream until stiff and add this (or 4 ounces of the non-dairy whipped substitute) to the mixture.

Fold this creamed mixture into the sponge cake bits. Pour gently into the prepared pan. Refrigerate for several hours or overnight.

To serve, reverse entire springform pan onto a large plate or tray. Carefully remove sides and bottom of pan. Cut into wedges and serve plain with the remaining 1 cup whipped cream, whipped with the rum and sugar. Top with sliced berries. *Makes 12 servings.*

NOTE: You may substitute leftover sponge or angel food cake for the sponge roll.

PUDDINGS

CREAMY RICE PUDDING

A melt-in-your-mouth pudding, good enough for a company dessert when topped with a dab of whipped cream and a maraschino cherry.

4 cups whole milk or
    nondairy liquid
$^1/_2$ cup white rice,
    uncooked
$^1/_2$ teaspoon salt
$^1/_3$ cup sugar
3 egg whites
1 egg yolk

$^1/_2$ cup golden raisins
1 teaspoon dried orange
    peel
2 teaspoons vanilla
Whipped cream, for
    topping (optional)
6 maraschino cherries

In a 2-quart saucepan, over medium heat, bring 3 cups of the milk, the rice, and salt to a boil. Reduce heat to low. Cover pan and simmer for about 35 minutes, or until the milk is almost absorbed and the rice is tender. Stir frequently.

With an electric mixer, beat the sugar, egg whites, and yolk for about a minute or until very frothy. Add the last cup of milk and beat for a couple of seconds. Mix this, the raisins, orange peel, and vanilla into the warm cooked rice.

Cook over low heat, stirring constantly, until the pudding is hot and thickened, about 7 to 8 minutes. Cool, cover, and refrigerate. Serve in sherbet dishes topped with whipped cream and a maraschino cherry, if desired. *Makes 5 or 6 servings.*

SPICY BREAD PUDDING

A creamy bread custard filled with spices to make this a taste treat and a good way to use up bread or cookie crumbs.

1 scant cup dry GF bread or cookie crumbs	1/8 teaspoon salt
2 cups rich milk, scalded	1 tablespoon butter, melted
1/3 cup sugar	2 eggs, beaten slightly
1/2 teaspoon Chinese-style five-spice seasoning (see Note)	1/2 cup dried fruit, chopped, or golden raisins
1 teaspoon dried orange peel	Cream or whipped cream, for topping

Preheat oven to 350°.

Soak the bread crumbs in the scalded milk for 5 minutes. Add the sugar, five-spice seasoning, orange peel, salt, and butter. Slowly blend in the eggs and stir. Add the chopped fruit. Pour the custard into a greased 2-quart dish and place the casserole in a shallow pan of hot water. Bake for about 1 hour, or until firm. Serve either hot or cold with cream or whipped cream. *Makes 4 servings.*

This recipe can easily be doubled, in which case use a 3-quart casserole for baking.

NOTE: Chinese-style five-spice seasoning can be found in the spice or oriental section of most large grocery stores. If unavailable, substitute a dash each of cinnamon, cloves, and nutmeg.

APPLE PUDDING

A moist, rich, fruity English-style pudding. This has the flavor of apple pie with the addition of nuts and currants. If desired, top it with ice cream or rum-flavored whipped cream (see page 180). It is best served warm, but can be made ahead and rewarmed.

1/2 cup dried currants	3 whole eggs
3 tablespoons dark rum	3 egg yolks
4 cups cooking apples, peeled, cored, and minced	1/4 cup GF flour mix
	2 teaspoons baking powder
	1/2 cup apple juice
1/2 cup brown sugar	1 cup rich cream or nondairy liquid
1 teaspoon cinnamon	
2 tablespoons lemon juice	2 teaspoons vanilla
4 tablespoons (1/2 stick) butter or margarine	1/2 cup chopped walnuts or pecans
1/2 cup granulated sugar	Dash salt

Preheat oven to 325°.

In a small saucepan, heat together the currants and rum until just warm. Set aside.

Tumble the apples with the brown sugar, cinnamon, and lemon juice. In a heavy frying pan, heat the butter and add the spiced apples. Sauté until the apples are tender, about 10 minutes. Set aside.

In a large mixing bowl, beat together the sugar, eggs, and egg yolks until fluffy.

Sift together the flour and baking powder; beat into the yolk mixture. Add the apple juice, cream, and vanilla. Beat until smooth. Stir in the cooked apple mixture, currants in rum, and nuts. Add the salt and pour into a greased 2-quart casserole or soufflé dish. Bake until pudding is set, about 1 hour and 25 minutes.

Serve while warm topped with ice cream or Rum-Flavored Whipped Cream, if desired. *Serves 6 to 8.*

RUM-FLAVORED WHIPPED CREAM

To 1 cup whipping cream whipped, add 1 tablespoon sugar, 1 tablespoon dark rum, and 1 teaspoon vanilla.

RHUBARB FOOL

A fruit custard dish from my mother's family recipes, but I've replaced her rich cream with yogurt. It is easy to make and calls for few ingredients.

2¹/₂ cups rhubarb (³/₄ pound; see Note)	3 tablespoons orange juice
¹/₂ cup sugar	1 teaspoon cornstarch
¹/₂ teaspoon dried orange peel (see Note)	¹/₂ teaspoon vanilla
	1 cup yogurt

In a medium saucepan, combine the rhubarb, sugar, orange peel, and 2 tablespoons of the orange juice. Simmer, covered, for 5 minutes.

In a small bowl, stir together the remaining tablespoon of orange juice and the cornstarch. Pour into the rhubarb mixture. Cook, stirring, until thickened and bubbly. Cool.

Just before serving, stir the vanilla into the yogurt and fold this into the rhubarb mixture. *Makes 4 servings.*

NOTE: If fresh rhubarb is unavailable, use a frozen 12-ounce package.

Fresh orange zest may be used instead of dried orange peel, in which case add 1 to 1¹/₂ teaspoons after, instead of during, cooking.

APPETIZERS

CRACKERS, GRANOLA, AND PRETZELS

Sesame Thins
Pecan Wafers
Corn Chips
Italian Cheese Straws
Cheese Crisps
Light Granola
  Light Granola Bars
Pretzels

MEAT, FISH, OR CHEESE HORS D'OEUVRES

Shanghai Chicken Wings
Indonesian Meatballs with
  Pineapple Sauce
Norwegian Fish Balls
Beef or Pork Sâté

Chicken or Pork Sâté
Chinese Egg Rolls
Potato Nachos

PÂTÉS AND SPREADS

Easy Salmon Pâté
  Salmon Dip

DIPS AND SAUCES

Double Dill Dip
Tartar Sauce
Peanut Sauce
Sweet Mustard Sauce

SEE ALSO

Hawaiian Chicken Chunks
Grandma's Chicken Wings
Mediterranean Meatballs

Appetizers, *pupus*, or hors d'oeuvres—whatever they're called around the world—may be a tasty addition to parties, but for the celiac they are merely another frustration. The crackers contain wheat; so does the bread. And most of the lovely nibbles have gluten in the filling, sauce, or seasoning. The fruit slices are safe and so are the veggies, but watch the dip.

Since many receptions and openings often serve only appetizers, I used to carry my dull (but safe) little rice crackers in my purse—something to eat with that obligatory glass of white wine or seltzer.

Now all that has changed. I can have crackers that look like the ones served, and they taste good, too. I have included these cracker recipes in this section, along with recipes (revised to gluten free) for some of the most interesting hors d'oeuvres from faraway lands—sâtés of Singapore, fish balls from Norway, nachos from Mexico, and Shanghai teriyaki chicken wings.

Next time you browse a table of hors d'oeuvres, just pull out your own tasty crackers to nibble with the wine and think of all those gluten-free appetizers you can make at home for your guests—and yourself.

CRACKERS, GRANOLA, AND PRETZELS

SESAME THINS

Delicious gluten-free crackers to eat with cheese, dips, or just plain, these are easy to make and keep crisp for several weeks if stored in a closed container. (If you wish to keep these longer, freeze them.)

1/2 cup brown rice flour (coarse)
1/2 cup GF flour mix
1/2 teaspoon xanthan gum
1 teaspoon baking powder
1/4 teaspoon salt
3 tablespoons margarine

2 tablespoons dark corn syrup
2 tablespoons toasted sesame seeds
2 to 4 tablespoons rich milk or nondairy liquid

Preheat oven to 350°.

In a medium mixing bowl, combine the rice flour, GF flour mix, xanthan gum, baking powder, and salt. Add the margarine and corn syrup and mix until the dough feels like coarse crumbs. Stir in the sesame seeds. Add milk gradually, using just enough to form a ball.

Roll out the dough on a rice-floured board to 1/8 inch (or less) thick. Cut with a pastry wheel into 1 1/2-by-1 1/2-inch squares. Using a spatula, transfer to ungreased cookie sheets. Bake for 10 to 12 minutes, or until firm and toasted looking. The thinner the cracker, the less time in the oven. *Makes 3 dozen.*

PECAN WAFERS

A thin party wafer with a nutty crunch, excellent eaten alone, with cream cheese, or used as a base for a meat or fish spread. This is another easily made cracker that keeps for weeks in an airtight container.

3/4 cup rice cream cereal (uncooked; see Note)
3/4 cup GF flour mix
3/4 teaspoon xanthan gum
1 1/2 teaspoons baking powder
1/2 teaspoon salt

4 1/2 tablespoons margarine
3 tablespoons light corn syrup
3 tablespoons finely ground pecans
3 to 4 tablespoons rich milk or nondairy liquid

Preheat oven to 350°.

In a medium mixing bowl, combine the cereal, GF flour mix, xanthan gum, baking powder, and salt. Add the margarine and corn syrup and mix until dough feels like coarse crumbs. Stir in the pecans. Add milk gradually, using just enough for the dough to form a ball.

Roll the dough on a rice-floured board to 1/8 inch thick. Cut with a pastry wheel into 1 1/2-by-1 1/2-inch squares. Bake on ungreased cookie sheets for 10 to 12 minutes, or until firm. *Makes 4 1/2 dozen.*

NOTE: Brown Rice Cream cereal or Pacific Rice's Quick 'n Creamy are in health food stores and some grocery stores. If unavailable, use 1/4 cup brown rice and 1/2 cup Cream of Rice cereal.

CORN CHIPS

This chip is baked, not deep-fried like most corn chips on the market, thus eliminating much of the fat. These are easily made and have a fine corn flavor delicately spiced with orange. The crackers keep for several weeks in an airtight container, or they may be frozen for later use.

3/4 cup quick hominy
   grits
3/4 cup GF flour mix
3/4 teaspoon xanthan gum
1/2 teaspoon salt
11/2 teaspoons baking
   powder

1 teaspoon dried orange
   peel
3 tablespoons light corn
   syrup
41/2 tablespoons margarine
3 to 4 tablespoons rich
   milk or nondairy liquid

Preheat oven to 350°.

In a medium mixing bowl, combine the grits, GF flour mix, xanthan gum, salt, baking powder, and orange peel. Add the corn syrup and margarine and mix until dough feels like coarse crumbs. Add the milk gradually, using just enough for the dough to form a ball.

Roll out on a rice-floured board to 1/8 inch or less thick. Cut with a pastry wheel into 11/2-by-11/2-inch squares. Transfer with spatula to ungreased cookie sheets. Bake for 10 to 12 minutes, or until firm and toasted looking. *Makes 41/2 dozen chips.*

ITALIAN CHEESE STRAWS

A great, flaky appetizer stick for parties or just munching, this is doubly cheesy; there is cheese in the dough and more in the topping.

Pastry

1¹/₂ cups white rice flour
¹/₂ cup tapioca flour
1 teaspoon baking powder
1 teaspoon xanthan gum
1 teaspoon salt
1 cup (2 sticks) margarine,
  melted
¹/₂ cup ricotta cheese

¹/₂ cup sour cream
  (no substitute)

Topping

1 egg, beaten slightly
²/₃ cup grated Parmesan
  cheese
1 tablespoon paprika

In a medium mixing bowl, blend together the flours, baking powder, xanthan gum, and salt. Stir in the margarine. Add the ricotta cheese and sour cream. The dough will look more like cooked cereal than pastry. Chill for 2 hours, or until the dough becomes firm and easy to handle.

Preheat oven to 400°.

Divide the dough into thirds and roll out each section on a rice-floured board to a thickness of a little over ¹/₈ inch (it's easier if you place plastic wrap on top of the dough). Brush with beaten egg and sprinkle on the cheese and paprika. Cut into strips ¹/₂ inch by 4 inches. Bake on an ungreased cookie sheet for 10 to 12 minutes, or until well browned. Cool. Store in an airtight container in the refrigerator. *Makes 4 to 5 dozen straws.*

CHEESE CRISPS

Finally! A successful cheese cracker for snacking, spreading, and dipping.

1¹/₂ cups white rice flour
¹/₂ cup tapioca flour
1 teaspoon baking powder
1 teaspoon xanthan gum
1 teaspoon salt
²/₃ cup grated Parmesan
   cheese

1 tablespoon paprika
1 cup (2 sticks) margarine,
   melted
¹/₂ cup ricotta cheese
¹/₂ cup sour cream

In a medium mixing bowl, blend together the flours, baking powder, xanthan gum, salt, Parmesan cheese, and paprika. Add the margarine, ricotta cheese, and sour cream. The dough will resemble cooked cereal. Chill for 2 hours until the dough becomes firm and easy to handle.

Preheat oven to 400°.

Divide the dough into thirds and roll out each section on a rice-floured board to a thickness resembling pastry dough (it's easier if you place plastic wrap on top of the dough). Prick overall with a fork. Cut with pastry wheel into 1¹/₂-by-1¹/₂-inch squares (or the size you wish). Transfer to ungreased cookie sheets and bake for 8 to 10 minutes. Watch them to keep them from browning too much. The thinner they are, the less time they'll need. Cool and store in airtight containers in the refrigerator. *Makes 6 dozen crackers.*

LIGHT GRANOLA

I've found this less-sweet version of my original granola a completely satisfying breakfast; it provides protein, fiber, and fruit. There is no need to add sugar, for there is sweetness in the coating. It's great also for snacking, carrying on trips, topping yogurt, including in bread (see Swiss Granola Bread, page 48). Try also the Light Granola Bars on page 190. (Double the recipe if more than one person is eating the cereal, and it will still stay fresh tasting to the end.)

3 cups GF puffed rice
3 cups GF cornflakes,
 crushed
1 cup Perky's Nutty Rice
 cereal
1 cup roasted soy nuts,
 peanuts, coconut, pine
 nuts, or almonds
1 cup sunflower seeds
1/2 teaspoon salt (if nuts
 and sunflower seeds are
 unsalted)

1/4 cup honey
1/4 cup vegetable oil
1 cup raisins or dried
 currants
1 cup of any of the
 following: dried peach
 or apricot bits, dried
 date bits, dried banana
 flakes, dried cherries or
 apples, dried pineapple

Preheat oven to 225°.

Coat a large roaster with GF vegetable spray. Put in the cereals, nuts, seeds, and salt (if used).

In a small saucepan, combine the honey and oil. Heat to boiling, stirring constantly since this mixture has a tendency to foam over the minute it comes to a boil. Remove from heat and drizzle over the mixture in the roaster. Stir well.

Bake for 2 hours, stirring every 30 minutes to keep the mixture from sticking together. Add the raisins and fruit and turn off the oven to cool down. The granola will be okay if left overnight.

Store granola in a plastic container. *Makes about 10 cups or enough for 2 batches of granola bars.*

NOTE: This basic recipe can be varied as your imagination dictates or according to supplies on the kitchen shelf. Add Kenmai Rice Bran, chopped popcorn, and dried orange or lemon peel for additional flavoring.

LIGHT GRANOLA BARS

Here is a less-sweet version of my original granola bars.

2 tablespoons brown sugar
1/4 cup dark corn syrup
1/3 cup sweetened
   condensed milk
2 tablespoons butter or
   margarine, melted

1/2 teaspoon vanilla
   flavoring or dried lemon
   peel
4 1/2 cups granola mixture,
   chopped coarsely in a
   food processor

Preheat oven to 350°.

In a medium bowl, combine the brown sugar, corn syrup, milk, margarine, and vanilla. Pour over the granola and mix thoroughly. This will be sticky. Butter hands and pat mixture into a greased 9" × 13" pan. Bake for 20 minutes. Cool for about 10 minutes and then cut into bars. If left longer, they will be hard to cut. Store in airtight containers for 2 to 3 weeks. The flavor improves with age. *Makes about twenty 1 1/2-by-3-inch chewy bars.*

PRETZELS

Have you been hungering for a pretzel? Why not make your own? Great for parties and perfect as nibbles when traveling by car or boat, for they settle a motion-disturbed stomach. These keep well but may become hard. Don't throw them out; just dunk them in your coffee or drink.

1 recipe Rapid-Rise French Bread batter (page 41)
1 egg white, slightly beaten
Coarse sea salt

Preheat oven to 400°.

Mix up the recipe for French Bread. Place the dough immediately in a plastic bag with a 1/4-inch opening cut from one corner. Squeeze out into pretzel shapes on 2 or more greased cookie sheets, leaving an inch between pretzels for rising.

Brush lightly with the slightly beaten egg white and sprinkle on the salt. Let rise for 25 minutes.

Bake for about 10 minutes, or until the pretzels are dry and toasty brown. When cool, transfer to a plastic bag or airtight container. *Makes 8 dozen 2-inch pretzels.*

MEAT, FISH, OR CHEESE HORS D'OEUVRES

SHANGHAI CHICKEN WINGS

These tasty chicken wings baked in a sweet marinade sauce may be served in the sauce or drained and reheated for easier eating. Look for the prepackaged chicken wings in either the frozen food section or the fresh meat counter. If the wings are whole, cut off the bony tips and cut each wing into two pieces.

2 1/2 pounds chicken wings	1 tablespoon fresh grated gingerroot
2 cups chicken broth	1/4 cup dry white wine or 7UP
1 cup brown sugar	
1/4 cup granulated sugar	1/4 cup GF soy sauce

Preheat oven to 400°.

Rinse and pat the chicken dry.

In a medium size bowl, mix together the broth, sugars, ginger, wine, and soy sauce.

Place the chicken wings in 9″ × 11″ pan or casserole. Pour on the marinade. Let set for 1 hour, and bake for 45 minutes.

Serve immediately, or remove from the sauce, reserving it, and store overnight to reheat the next day. Brush lightly with the sauce before heating. *Serves 8 to 10 as an appetizer.*

INDONESIAN MEATBALLS WITH PINEAPPLE SAUCE

An appetizer meatball with a subtle blend of Far East flavors. Serve it in Pineapple Sauce, below, or with a selection of spicy sauces found on pages 199 and 200, and let your guests dip as they choose. These freeze well so can be made weeks ahead.

²/₃ pound lean ground beef	2 tablespoons GF soy sauce
¹/₃ pound lean ground pork	¹/₄ teaspoon garlic salt
¹/₃ cup GF bread crumbs or GF cereal, crushed	1 egg
1¹/₂ teaspoons curry powder	1 tablespoon dry milk powder
1 tablespoon peanut butter	1 teaspoon prepared mustard
Salt and pepper to taste	1 tablespoon sesame or peanut oil, for frying
¹/₂ teaspoon ginger	Pineapple Sauce (see page 193)

Preheat oven to 350°.

In a large bowl, mix together all the ingredients except the oil. Form into ³/₄-inch balls. Heat the oil in a heavy skillet and brown the balls, about a dozen at a time, shaking the skillet to keep them round. Cook only until the balls are browned and crusty. Remove the meatballs to a baking dish and fry the next batch.

When all the balls are done, bake for about 45 minutes, covered with the Pineapple Sauce, if desired. Or bake plain and serve with dipping sauces on the side. Provide toothpicks for your guests. *Serves 8 to 10 as an appetizer.*

PINEAPPLE SAUCE

1 cup pineapple juice	1 teaspoon grated fresh
2 tablespoons cornstarch	gingerroot
2 tablespoons lime juice	1/4 cup sake, dry white
1/3 cup brown sugar	wine, or 7UP

Put the pineapple juice in a small saucepan. In a bowl, blend together the cornstarch, lime juice, brown sugar, and ginger. Add to the pineapple juice. Cook until clear and slightly thickened. Remove from heat and add wine or 7UP. Pour over the meatballs before baking.

NORWEGIAN FISH BALLS

Tiny and tender deep-fried fish balls add a different taste to the hors d'oeuvres table. Serve with picks and offer a dipping sauce to add to the flavor. The fish balls can be made ahead and frozen. Thaw on the day of the party and then microwave or reheat in a 350° oven just before the guests arrive.

1 1/2 pounds bottom fish,	1/8 teaspoon mace
fresh or frozen (cod,	2/3 cup evaporated milk or
halibut, snapper)	fresh nondairy liquid
1 small onion	3/4 teaspoon salt
1 egg	Oil, for deep-frying
1 1/2 tablespoons potato	Suggested sauces: Double
starch flour	Dill Dip and Tartar
1/4 teaspoon pepper	Sauce (page 199)
1/4 teaspoon nutmeg	

Wash and remove any bones and skin from the fish. Place the fish and onion in a food processor fitted with metal blade and process until thoroughly pulped.

Transfer to a mixing bowl and, with electric mixer, beat in the egg, flour, pepper, nutmeg, and mace. Gradually add the milk, beating until the mixture is light and fluffy, about 15 minutes. Stir in the salt.

Heat 2 inches of oil in deep-fat fryer or a deep heavy pan. Drop 3/4-to-1-inch rounds of the batter from a wet melon baller (or the tip of a teaspoon) into the hot oil until the balls are brown and crusty with a very moist center. Drain on paper toweling. Transfer to a serving casserole to be reheated, or cool and freeze for later use. *Makes 10 dozen balls.*

BEEF OR PORK SÂTÉ

Earn raves with this appetizer! I first saw these meat-on-a-skewer snacks served in open restaurants on Singapore streets. Now they appear on many buffets. The strong garlic flavor is especially good with beef. Although a little troublesome to make, this hors d'oeuvre can be prepared and broiled ahead of time.

2 pounds sirloin steak or pork tenderloin	2 tablespoons brown sugar
2 teaspoons finely chopped garlic	Thirty 4-inch bamboo skewers
2 teaspoons salt	2 tablespoons peanut oil, for brushing
1/4 teaspoon pepper	Peanut Sauce (page 200) or
1/2 cup GF soy sauce	Sweet Mustard Sauce
1/4 cup lime juice	(page 200), for dipping

Slice the meat into 1/8-inch-thick strips. Set aside.

In a small bowl, combine the garlic, salt, and pepper. Mash the mixture into a paste. Transfer it to a large bowl and add the soy sauce, lime juice, and brown sugar. Add the meat strips and toss until evenly coated. Let marinate for 2 hours in the refrigerator, turning occasionally.

Meanwhile, soak the bamboo skewers in water to prevent burning while broiling.

Thread the meat on the soaked skewers, packing it tightly with about 1/2 inch of wood sticking out of each end. Place about half the skewers in a single layer on vegetable oil–sprayed foil in a 9″ × 13″ baking pan. Brush with oil.

At this point you may refrigerate them for later broiling the same day, or do as I do: broil now, then refrigerate, and reheat later. Broil the first side about 5 inches from heat for about 5 minutes. Turn and broil for 4 to 5 minutes on the other side, or until the meat is browned. Serve immediately—or remove to a large casserole and broil the second batch.

You may freeze or refrigerate these overnight. About 30 minutes before party time, reheat, covered, in a 375° oven. Serve with one of the sauces. *Makes 30 sâtés.*

CHICKEN OR PORK SÂTÉ

A different and milder sâté from Beef or Pork Sâté. I served both at a party, thinking I would put the most popular in this book. My guests insisted both should be included.

1 1/2 pounds boneless
   chicken breast or pork
   tenderloin
2 teaspoons fresh grated
   gingerroot
1 1/4 cups coconut milk
3 teaspoons ginger-curry
   powder

1/4 teaspoon salt
Twenty-four 4-inch
   bamboo skewers
Sweet Mustard Sauce (page
   200) or Peanut Sauce
   (page 200), for dipping

Wash the chicken or pork and slice into thin strips. Set aside.

In a large bowl, mix the gingerroot, coconut milk, ginger-curry powder, and salt. Add the meat strips and toss gently. Marinate in the refrigerator for 1 hour or more.

Place the bamboo skewers in water to soak.

Thread the meat on the soaked skewers, packing tightly with 1/2 inch of wood left at each end. Place skewers in a single layer on a vegetable oil–sprayed foil in a 9″ × 13″ baking pan.

At this point you may refrigerate them for later broiling the same day, or broil now, then refrigerate, and reheat later. Broil the first side about 5 inches from heat for about 5 minutes. Turn and broil the other side for about 4 minutes, or until the meat is browned. Serve immediately—or refrigerate. These also freeze well. About 30 minutes before party time, reheat, covered, in preheated 375° oven. Serve with one of the sauces. *Makes about 24 sâtés.*

CHINESE EGG ROLLS

We can't eat egg rolls in a restaurant but we can make them at home. They are a bit of trouble, but well worth it. I've given the filling ingredients plus instructions for two ways of wrapping these. Use edible rice paper found in oriental stores, or for an easier method, form the rolls and dip them in Tempura Batter before deep-frying.

1 cup chopped cooked
  chicken or shrimp
1/2 cup fresh bean sprouts,
  chopped
One 8-ounce can water
  chestnuts, drained and
  chopped
One 8-ounce can bamboo
  shoots, drained and
  chopped
3 green onions, chopped

1/4 cup chopped green bell
  pepper (for shrimp roll
  only)
1 teaspoon fresh grated
  gingerroot
1/4 cup ground almonds
2 teaspoons GF soy sauce
1 egg, beaten
Vegetable oil, for frying
12 pieces rice paper, or
  Tempura Batter
  (page 249)

Mix together all ingredients except the egg, oil, and rice paper.

For the rice paper method, spread about 1 large tablespoon of the filling down the center of each piece of rice paper, which handles better when kept slightly moist. Fold side edges over filling, then roll carefully in jelly roll fashion. Seal the open edge with the egg. Place fold side down and allow to dry before frying. Fry in hot 360° oil until brown. If you don't have a gauge on your fryer, test the oil by dropping in a one-inch cube of bread. It should brown in 60 seconds. *Makes 12 rolls.* Cut in 1¹/₂-inch sections to serve.

Tempura method: Make one batch of the tempura batter. Instead of using the beaten egg for sealing, put it into the filling mixture as a binder. Moisten your hands and form small rolls (about 1 by 3 inches). Then, using a slotted spoon, dip them into the tempura batter and then lower into the hot oil. Cook until brown and crusty. *Makes about 14 rolls.*

POTATO NACHOS

A delicious change from the corn chip nachos, Potato Nachos have no oil. I suggest Cheez Whiz, but always check to see that it is still gluten free.

6 medium potatoes
Salt and pepper to taste
One 8-ounce jar Mild
   Mexican Cheez Whiz
2 tablespoons thinly sliced
   green onions

One 2¹/₂-ounce can sliced
   black olives, drained
1 cup sour cream or
   nondairy substitute

Preheat oven to 375°.

Scrub the potatoes and cut into thin slices. Place in a single layer on greased cookie sheets, sprinkle with salt and pepper, and bake for 25 to 30 minutes, or until crisp and lightly browned.

Pile the hot chips on a large serving plate. Heat the cheese spread according to directions and pour over the potatoes. Sprinkle on the green onion and black olives. Top with sour cream. Serve immediately. *Makes 6 servings.*

PÂTÉS AND SPREADS

EASY SALMON PÂTÉ

A quick and easy appetizer spread, with a fresher taste than purchased ones. Stir this up a few hours before guests arrive. Serve with any of the appetizer crackers in this section or make the Pumpernickel or Russian Black Bread (pages 44 and 42) in small loaves and slice to serve as crackers.

One 7½-ounce can salmon	⅓ cup mayonnaise
One 3-ounce package	1 tablespoon lemon juice
cream cheese	1 tablespoon grated onion

Drain the salmon, reserving juice for thinning if necessary. Pick off the skin or dark pieces.

Soften the cream cheese and blend in the mayonnaise, lemon juice, and onion. Stir in the salmon. Place in a serving bowl and chill. *Makes about 1¼ cups.*

SALMON DIP: Prepare as above, adding enough of the reserved juice to make desired dipping consistency. Top with fresh minced parsley just before serving. *Makes about 1½ cups.*

DIPS AND SAUCES

DOUBLE DILL DIP

Great for vegetables or the Norwegian Fish Balls (page 193), Double Dill Dip is simple to make and doubly flavorful. I use Uncle Dan's Country Dill dressing and dip mix for this, but you may find a different one on your grocery shelf. Be sure to read labels to confirm that your mix is gluten free.

1 cup sour cream or nondairy substitute	1 package GF dried dill dressing and dip mix
1 cup mayonnaise	1 teaspoon dried dill weed

Blend together the sour cream and mayonnaise. Add the dressing mix and dill weed. Cover and refrigerate for at least 24 hours to achieve maximum flavor. *Makes 1 pint.*

TARTAR SAUCE

You can stir up this quick tartar sauce for a dip or to serve with vegetables or fish. GF sweet pickles can be found at some health food stores or, to be safe, make your own during cucumber season (see pages 252 and 253).

1 cup mayonnaise	1 tablespoon chopped fresh parsley
2 tablespoons GF sweet pickles, minced	1 teaspoon lemon juice
1 tablespoon chopped green olives	1 tablespoon grated onion

Place mayonnaise in a bowl. Add the other ingredients and stir well. Cover and refrigerate to let flavors meld for several hours before serving. *Makes about 1 cup.*

PEANUT SAUCE

A sâté is incomplete without a dipping sauce. This is great for the Beef Sâté on page 194. It can be made ahead and reheated just before serving. If it seems too thick, thin with more chicken stock or hot water.

2 tablespoons vegetable oil
1/4 cup finely chopped
   green onions (white part
   only)
1 teaspoon finely chopped
   garlic
One 14-ounce can chicken
   stock

1/2 cup creamy peanut
   butter
1 1/2 tablespoons GF soy
   sauce
1 teaspoon lime juice
1 1/2 teaspoons fresh grated
   gingerroot
3 to 4 drops Tabasco sauce

In a heavy 2-quart saucepan, heat the oil and sauté the onion and garlic for 3 or 4 minutes, until they are translucent. Pour in the chicken stock and bring it to a boil over high heat. Stirring constantly, add the peanut butter, soy sauce, lime juice, ginger, and Tabasco. Reduce heat to low and simmer for about 10 minutes, stirring occasionally. The sauce should thicken some. Serve hot in bowls suitable for dipping the sâtés. *Makes about 2 cups.*

SWEET MUSTARD SAUCE

One of my most popular dipping sauces—and the easiest. Use this for the Beef or Pork Sâté (page 194) or the Chicken or Pork Sâté (page 195).

1/2 cup grape or currant jelly
1/2 cup prepared mustard

Heat the jelly and mustard together in a small saucepan over medium heat, stirring frequently, until the jelly is melted and the sauce is hot. Do not boil or overheat. Pour immediately into a bowl suitable for dipping the sâté. *Makes 1 cup.*

SOUPS

CREAM SOUPS
Asparagus Soup
Curried Cream of Tomato
  Soup
  Crab or Lobster Bisque
Easy Cream of Chicken
  Soup

CHOWDERS
Fresh Corn Chowder
Polish Potato Chowder

BEAN SOUPS
Greek Bean Soup
Navy Bean Soup, Yankee
  Style

Portuguese Vegetable Soup
  with Kidney Beans

SPECIALTY SOUPS
Gazpacho
French Onion Soup
Japanese Chicken-Noodle
  Soup

SEE ALSO
Creamed Soup Base
Onion Soup Mix

If it's soup for lunch (or dinner), the celiac or wheat-allergic person soon discovers one can seldom open a can or packet. That lovely collection of soups on the grocery shelves usually contains gluten in the form of pasta, barley, or wheat for thickening. Even the vegetable soups may be started with a base of gluten-laced bouillon.

As in most of our cooking, it's back to scratch. That's not all bad, for homemade soups are far more tasty and nutritious than commercial soups. Only since I started making my own soups have I begun to enjoy them as complete meals.

The recipes on the following pages cover tastes for every palate. Some, I hope, will become your favorites, as they have mine. I make them in large batches to pack in serving-sized freezer bags for several later meals. If you lay the bags flat while freezing, they take little room and defrost easily. One visitor, who admitted his wife was a can-opener cook, upon seeing my collection of frozen soup, remarked, "Gosh, look at that. You could live for a year without opening a can."

Not quite. But I can have a great meal of thick soup on the table while my home-baked (frozen) bread is defrosting. So can you with a bit of extra planning.

For a handy ready-made soup mix when a recipe calls for canned soup, see the Creamed Soup Base on page 335.

CREAM SOUPS

ASPARAGUS SOUP

Mild and creamy with the gentle flavor of spring, this may be used as a soup or as a sauce to flavor chicken and pork casseroles. It is easy to make because you use canned asparagus, but if you prefer a cream-colored sauce—one tester said her children didn't like the pale green appearance—use French or blanched asparagus.

One 10-ounce can cut asparagus (see Note)
4 tablespoons sweet rice flour
1 teaspoon salt (or to taste)
1/2 teaspoon pepper (white preferred)

4 cups chicken broth
1 teaspoon onion powder
1/2 teaspoon garlic powder
One 12-ounce can evaporated milk or nondairy liquid

Drain the asparagus, reserving liquid. Blend pieces in a blender.

Pour the blended asparagus into a large saucepan. Add the flour, salt, and pepper. Slowly stir in the reserved liquid and the chicken broth. Add the onion and garlic powders. Cook for a short while and then add the evaporated milk. Cook over medium heat, stirring constantly, until thickened slightly to a thin cream soup texture. Serve warm. *Makes 6 servings.*

NOTE: You may substitute one 10-ounce package of frozen asparagus, cooked according to package directions.

CURRIED CREAM OF
TOMATO SOUP

A delicate touch of curry spices up an old favorite. This quick and easy soup can be served hot or cold. For a heartier soup, add crab or lobster (see below).

4 tablespoons butter or margarine, divided	1 teaspoon curry powder
2 cups tomatoes, peeled and diced	2 tablespoons white rice flour
1 medium onion, diced	1 1/2 cups rich milk or nondairy liquid
Salt and pepper to taste	

In a medium saucepan, melt 2 tablespoons of the butter. Add the tomatoes, onion, dash of salt and pepper. Bring to a boil and then simmer, covered, for about 10 minutes, or until the onions are clear. Remove to a blender and puree.

In the same saucepan, melt the rest of the butter. Stir in the curry powder and rice flour and immediately add the milk. Cook until thickened.

Return the pureed tomato mixture to the thickened sauce. Season to taste with salt and pepper and heat. Serve immediately or refrigerate to serve cold. *Makes 4 servings.*

CRAB OR LOBSTER BISQUE: A super soup and so easy! Add at the final heating one 6 1/2-ounce can crab or lobster or 1/2 cup fresh crab or lobster. Serve hot topped with your choice of grated Cheddar cheese or chopped fresh parsley. *Makes 4 to 6 servings.*

EASY CREAM OF
CHICKEN SOUP

I created this in desparation when the doctor put me on a soft-food diet. Since then, I've found many uses for this quick and easy cream soup. Use it for casseroles, as a topping for rice or potatoes, or take it in the Thermos as a hot dish for lunch.

One 5-ounce can chunky chicken	Salt to taste (optional)
2 cups chicken stock or 2 teaspoons chicken soup base (see Note) with 2 cups hot water	3 tablespoons rice flour
	2 tablespoons water
	1 cup milk or nondairy liquid

In a food processor, chop the chicken (plus liquid in can) into small chunks.

In a medium saucepan, place chopped chicken, chicken stock, and water. Bring to a boil. Salt to taste if necessary.

Blend together the rice flour and the water. Stir into the stock and cook until thickened. Add the milk and bring to the boiling point but don't boil. Remove from heat. *Makes 4 servings or approximately 4 cups soup to use in casserole dishes.* May be frozen.

NOTE: I use Crescent Chicken Soup Base, but there are other gluten-free brands on the market. Always read the ingredients list to be sure that your base is gluten free. If unavailable, substitute 2 cups chicken broth.

CHOWDERS

FRESH CORN CHOWDER

This soup, adapted from Bonnie S. Mickelson's recipe in Hollyhocks and Radishes, *is farm-fresh tasting and deliciously satisfying. Serve it with chunks of Rapid-Rise French Bread (page 41) for a full meal. Bonnie says the real flavor comes from freshly picked corn boiled only 3 minutes. Even though I tried this in midwinter and used frozen corn, it was still delicious. Canned whole kernel corn can also be used.*

1 cup onion, chopped fine	1/2 teaspoon dried basil
3 tablespoons butter or margarine	1/2 teaspoon dried sage, crushed
3/4 cup celery, chopped fine	2 cups chicken broth
2 tablespoons green or red bell pepper, diced	2 cups corn (about 4 ears) or 16 ounces frozen corn
1 1/2 cup cubed new potatoes	1 1/2 cups light cream plus 1/2 cup milk or 2 cups nondairy liquid
2 tablespoons rice flour	Salt and pepper to taste
1/2 teaspoon dried marjoram	Bacon bits and parsley, for garnish (optional)

In a large kettle, sauté the onion in butter until soft. Add the celery, bell pepper, and potatoes. Cook for 5 minutes, stirring often. Stir in the flour; cook 2 minutes longer. Add the marjoram, basil, sage, and chicken broth. Cover and simmer for 30 minutes, or until potatoes are tender.

Stir in the corn, cream, and milk. Add salt and pepper. Reheat but do not boil. Garnish, if desired, with the bacon bits and parsley. *Makes 6 servings.*

POLISH POTATO CHOWDER

This thick, rich, hearty soup with the extra vegetables and sausage is great when first made and even better the next day when the flavors have had a chance to blend. When reheated, it may need thinning. It's a quick and easy chowder.

2/3 to 1 pound Polish
   sausage
1/2 cup chopped onion
   (1/2 medium onion)
1/2 cup shredded carrot
2 tablespoons margarine or
   butter
2 cups sliced potatoes
   (3 medium)

1 1/2 cups chicken broth
1 cup milk or nondairy
   liquid
1 tablespoon rice flour
1/2 cup frozen peas
Salt and pepper to
   taste

If the sausage is cooked, dice it and set aside. If uncooked, cook fully, then dice.

In a large kettle or Dutch oven, sauté the onion and carrot in the margarine until soft. Add the potatoes and chicken broth. Simmer until potatoes are cooked, about 5 minutes. Mash them until no lumps appear.

Blend milk into the flour and add to the potato mixture. Bring to a boil and add the diced sausage. Heat through (do not boil) and add the frozen peas. Cook 2 minutes longer. Season with salt and pepper.

Serve immediately or cool and reheat later. *Makes 4 to 6 servings.*

BEAN SOUPS

GREEK BEAN SOUP

A Greek chef aboard a cruise ship shared his secret to this tasty soup: cook the vegetables the night before and soak the beans at the same time. The next evening you will have only an hour's cooking before dinner. For an even richer, tastier soup, add kielbasa sausage or cook a ham hock with the vegetables. Like many stews and soups, this is even better the next day. It also freezes well for another meal.

1/2 cup dry baby lima beans	2 cups celery, diced
1/2 cup dry pinto beans	1 cup carrots, diced
1/2 cup split peas (green or yellow)	2 cups beef broth (see Note)
9 cups water, divided	1 teaspoon dried thyme, crumbled
1 teaspoon salt	1/8 teaspoon red pepper
3 tablespoons butter or margarine	3/4 pound kielbasa sausage, sliced, or 1 1/2 pounds ham hock (optional; see Note)
1 medium onion, chopped	
1 large clove garlic, minced	

The night before: In a large bowl soak the lima beans, pinto beans, and split peas in 6 cups of the water with the salt. In a large Dutch oven or kettle, melt the butter. Sauté the onion, garlic, celery, and carrots for about 5 minutes, or until the onions are clear. Add the beef broth and 2 cups of the water. Simmer for 1 hour. Remove from heat and refrigerate overnight.

One hour (or more) before serving: Drain the beans and rinse. Add them plus 1 or more cups of water (to desired consistency) to the vegetable-beef broth. Add the thyme and red pepper. Bring to boil and simmer for 50 minutes or longer. If desired, add the sliced sausage during the last 15 minutes of cooking. *Makes 8 servings.*

NOTE: If using the ham hock, cook it with the vegetables and replace the 2 cups of beef broth with water. Leave it overnight; the next day, skin and bone the ham, chop the meat, and return it to the soup during the last 15 minutes of cooking.

NAVY BEAN SOUP, YANKEE STYLE

A great bean soup—hearty, delicious. This is good when first cooked but even better (as many soups are) the next day. It freezes well for later use. Remember the beans need to be presoaked. Many recipes for beans suggest boiling and then using the water in which the beans were boiled. I prefer the soaking and draining method suggested here to eliminate much of the gas often caused by the beans.

2 cups dried navy beans
1/3 cup vegetable oil
2 cloves garlic, minced
2 large onions, chopped
1/4 teaspoon thyme
One 5.5-ounce can
    V-8 juice
1 1/2 teaspoons salt
    (or to taste)

Pepper to taste
Boiling water as needed
1 1/2-pound ham hock
1 1/2 tablespoons lemon
    juice
2 tablespoons fresh
    parsley, minced, or
2 teaspoons dried
    parsley

Wash the beans and soak overnight in cold water. Drain and rinse.

Heat the oil in a large kettle or Dutch oven. Sauté the garlic and onions until clear. Add the beans, thyme, V-8 juice, salt, and pepper. Cover with enough water to come 2 inches above the beans.

Wash the ham hock and add it to the kettle.

Bring to boil and lower the heat. Cover and cook slowly until the beans are very soft and the ham falls from the bone, 2 1/2 to 3 hours. Remove ham bone and skin. Chop ham into bite-sized pieces and return it to the soup. To thicken, remove about 1 pint of beans and mash or pulverize them in a blender. Return to the kettle along with the lemon juice and parsley. Cook about 5 minutes longer. *Makes 8 servings.*

PORTUGUESE VEGETABLE SOUP
with Kidney Beans

A rich-flavored, hearty soup for those cold days, this one needs only bread or biscuits to make a meal. Then treat yourself to a dessert. Make ahead for extra flavor. Or make it and freeze some for another meal. For the sausage you may choose a "light" one and still have excellent flavor. Add pepper if you prefer more seasoning.

5 cups chicken broth
1 pound kielbasa sausage, diced
2 cups potato, peeled and diced
One 14-ounce can kidney beans, drained
One 14¹/₂-ounce can stewed tomatoes
1 cup chopped onions
1 cup diced carrots
¹/₂ head green cabbage, chopped
3 cloves garlic, minced

In a large soup pot, combine all the ingredients. Bring to a boil, stirring occasionally. Lower heat to a simmer and cook, stirring once in a while, for about 2 hours. Serve hot. *Makes 8 servings.*

SPECIALTY SOUPS

GAZPACHO

I assumed this cold vegetable soup from Spain was made of only vege-tables until I ate some and had a toxic reaction. Then I discovered that it often contains bread. The following version is not traditional but is flavorful and gluten free. The dab of sour cream for topping is purely an American touch and may be replaced with slices of avocado.

One 14½-ounce can
  whole peeled tomatoes
1½ cups chicken broth
2 tablespoons NutQuik,
  ground fine, or 12
  blanched almonds,
  ground
1½ teaspoons minced
  fresh parsley
1 small clove garlic,
  minced

1 small green bell pepper,
  seeded and chopped
1 cucumber, peeled
2 tablespoons olive oil
½ teaspoon salt
Dash cumin (optional)
One 5.5-ounce can
  V-8 juice
Sour cream or avocado
  slices, for topping

In a blender or food processor, puree the tomatoes. Remove and combine with the chicken broth.

In the blender, place the NutQuik, parsley, garlic, bell pepper, and cucumber. Blend until fine. Slowly add the olive oil, salt, cumin, and then part of the chicken broth–tomato mixture.

Remove from blender and add the remaining broth and the vege-table juice. Chill for at least 2 hours. Whisk just before serving. Garnish with your choice of sour cream or avocado slices. *Makes 4 or 5 servings.*

FRENCH ONION SOUP

An old favorite for the table and often called for in recipes, French Onion Soup can be served immediately or frozen in one-cup packets, then used when a casserole calls for onion soup. The recipe can easily be doubled. The French bread may be replaced with another GF bread, if desired.

1/4 cup (1/2 stick) butter or margarine	Dash pepper
2 to 3 large onions, sliced	1 teaspoon salt
3 1/2 cups beef broth	4 slices GF French Bread
1/2 cup dry sherry	(page 41; optional)
1 teaspoon Worcestershire sauce	1/2 to 3/4 cup grated Swiss cheese

In a large kettle, melt the butter and slowly cook the onions until translucent and slightly browned, about 20 minutes. Add the beef broth and sherry. Cover and simmer for 2 hours, stirring occasionally.

Near the end of the cooking time, add the Worcestershire sauce, pepper, and salt.

To serve, place each slice of bread, if desired, in the bottom of an individual ovenproof bowl. Fill bowls with soup. Top with a layer of grated cheese. Cook under the broiler until the cheese melts. Serve at once. *Makes 4 servings.*

JAPANESE CHICKEN-NOODLE SOUP

A friend confessed to me she was so hungry after hiking Mount Fuji that without realizing it she ate her noodle soup with chopsticks. The following soup is so thick and chunky you could do the same. This is a variation of the nábemono *(things in a pot) from Japan. It's a full-dish meal and has traditional Japanese visual appeal with a combination of colors and shapes. You may use homemade pasta (page 228) or purchased GF vermicelli.*

2 chicken breasts, boned
and skinned
1 egg white
1 tablespoon cornstarch
1 tablespoon sake or dry
white wine
4 cups chicken broth
1 cup water
2 teaspoons GF soy
sauce

3/4 cup uncooked GF
vermicelli
1 cup carrots, sliced
diagonally
6 Napa cabbage leaves, in
2-inch squares
6 green onions, in 1-inch
lengths
8 mushrooms, sliced
(shiitake or button)

Wash chicken breasts and slice into thin slivers; combine with the egg white, cornstarch, and sake. Set aside.

In a large kettle, bring the chicken broth, water, and soy sauce to boil. Break noodles to short lengths and add them to the broth. Cook for about 4 minutes. Add the carrots, cabbage, onions, and mushrooms. Cook until carrots are tender. Stir in the chicken and cook for 1 to 2 minutes. Serve Japanese style in deep bowls with large ceramic spoons. *Makes 4 or 5 servings.*

RICE, BEANS, AND PASTA

RICE

Singapore Rice Pot
Citrus Rice
Ginger Rice
Spiced Brown Rice
Curried Rice
   Curried Rice with Seafood
Vegetable Risotto with Tofu
Creamy Risotto with Apple
   and Cheese

BEANS AND LENTILS

Swedish Brown Beans
Hawaiian Pork and Beans
Butter-Basted Limas with
   Ham
Lentils Marrakesh (with
   Chicken)

PASTA

Fresh Egg Pasta
Fettuccine with Shrimp and
   Scallops
Touch-of-Irish Casserole
Savory Ham Casserole
   Chicken-Broccoli Supreme

KASHA

Lamb Kasha with Pine Nuts

SEE ALSO

Shrimp-Rice Pot
Deep Sea Delight
Sherried Chicken with Rice

Eating a mixed dish when dining out is dangerous for the celiac as there may be gluten in the thickening, flavoring, or bouillon, even if the base is supposedly gluten-free rice or beans. But what celiac or wheat-allergic person doesn't occasionally hunger for a crunchy casserole, a wonderful blend of favorite flavors?

The following pages of rice, bean, and pasta dishes should help appease that appetite—and likewise appeal to the thrifty cook, for most of them use little meat or the most inexpensive cuts. This selection was pared down to favorites as tried by my testers on their own families and guests.

The flavors cover a wide range, from a spicy rice pot to a tofu risotto. For the many tasty pasta dishes, you may make your own noodles from the Fresh Egg Pasta recipe or purchase GF pasta. There are more types of GF pasta on the market now; several of them do not need to be cooked with chicken and beef stock to be palatable and will not fall apart in casseroles. One that stands up especially well is the Drei Pauly brand, obtainable through Dietary Specialties, Inc. (see page 344). Warning for the soy intolerant: Many of these pastas include soy as one of the ingredients.

217

RICE

SINGAPORE RICE POT

From the crossroads of East and West comes this marvelously tasty blending of lamb, vegetables, and spiced rice. This dish takes but a short time to prepare and only one pot. Serve with a salad or fresh fruit plate for a full meal.

1 tablespoon vegetable oil	1 cup thin carrot slices
1 pound lean ground lamb	1/2 teaspoon salt
2/3 cup chopped onion	1 cup frozen peas, thawed
1 1/4 cups white rice	2 tablespoons minced
2 1/2 cups chicken stock	candied ginger
1/4 cup GF soy sauce	

Place a large heavy pot or Dutch oven over high heat, add the oil to coat the pan. Sauté the lamb and onion until the lamb browns slightly and the onion is translucent. Drain off extra grease.

Add the rice, chicken stock, soy sauce, carrots, and salt, and stir well. Bring to a boil, reduce heat, cover, and simmer for 20 to 25 minutes, or until liquid is absorbed. Stir occasionally. Add peas and sugared ginger and remove from heat to stand covered for 10 minutes before serving. *Makes 5 or 6 servings.*

CITRUS RICE

Rice with a delicate citrus flavor is a perfect accompaniment for any light-flavored fish or poultry. Slivered almonds may be substituted for the pine nuts, if desired.

2 tablespoons grated
   orange peel
1 teaspoon grated lime peel
1 teaspoon lemon peel
3/4 cup orange juice
2 tablespoons butter or
   margarine

1/4 cup chopped onion
1 cup white rice
1 1/4 cups water
1/2 teaspoon salt
1/4 cup pine nuts

In a 2 1/2- or 3-quart saucepan, heat the butter and sauté the onion until golden. Add the rice and stir until coated; pour in the juice, water, salt, and pine nuts. Add the peels. Bring to a boil. Reduce heat to a simmer and cook, covered, until rice is tender, about 20 to 25 minutes. *Makes 5 or 6 servings.*

GINGER RICE

Cashews, raisins, and curry spice up this rice into a couscouslike party dish. Serve it with chicken, ham, or pork and listen to your guests rave. I like this best with the nutty basmati rice but have also used white or brown rice.

2 1/4 cups chicken broth
1 cup rice
2 tablespoons lime juice
2 tablespoons crystalized
   ginger (minced)
2 tablespoons butter or
   margarine

1/2 teaspoon curry powder
1/2 cup golden raisins
1/3 cup coarsely chopped
   cashews
Salt to taste (optional)

In a 3-quart saucepan, bring the chicken broth to a boil. Stir in the rice, lime juice, minced ginger, butter, curry powder, raisins, and cashews. Salt to taste if the chicken broth is unsalted.

Cover, lower heat, and cook for 45 minutes for brown or basmati rice, or for about 20 minutes for white rice (or according to package directions), until the liquid has evaporated. This will be a moist dish. Serve while hot. *Makes 4 to 6 servings.*

SPICED BROWN RICE

I have transferred the spices and fruit of Moroccan couscous to brown rice and find the results excellent. For a completely Middle Eastern meal, serve this rice with the Moroccan Chicken (page 298). Or use it anytime you want a slightly sweet, seasoned rice full of fruit to offset simply cooked meat or poultry.

3 tablespoons butter or
  margarine
1 cup brown rice
2¼ cups chicken broth
¼ cup dried currants or
  raisins

¼ teaspoon salt, or to
  taste
⅛ teaspoon allspice
¼ teaspoon turmeric

In a large saucepan, heat the butter. Pour in the rice and stir to coat. Add the chicken broth, currants, salt, allspice, and turmeric. Bring to a boil. Stir once, then cover and lower heat to a simmer; cook for about 45 minutes, or according to the directions on the rice package, until the water is absorbed but the rice is still moist. *Makes 4 to 6 servings.*

CURRIED RICE

One of my favorites and so easy, this is a spicy rice-with-vegetable side dish wonderful with chicken, pork, or ham. It is mildly hot, but you can adjust the amount of curry powder to your taste. For a complete main dish, add cooked crabmeat and shrimp (see below).

6 tablespoons butter or margarine	2 teaspoons curry powder
1 cup onion, chopped	$1/8$ teaspoon cayenne pepper
1 cup celery, chopped	2 cups chicken broth
1 cup white rice	Salt and pepper to taste

In a large frying pan, melt the butter, add the onion and celery, and sauté, stirring occasionally, until onion is translucent.

Blend together the rice, curry powder, and cayenne pepper. Add to the onion mixture and stir while cooking until the rice is coated, about 2 minutes. Pour on the broth carefully. When it boils, cover pan and reduce heat to low. Simmer until rice is tender and the broth is absorbed, 18 to 20 minutes. Add salt and pepper to taste. *Makes 6 servings.*

CURRIED RICE WITH SEAFOOD: Proceed as for Curried Rice. After the rice is cooked, add $3/4$ cup either cooked crabmeat or GF imitation crabmeat or $3/4$ cup cooked, shelled shrimp, or a mix of the two, and 3 tablespoons minced parsley. Stir gently into the rice and heat for 5 minutes, or until seafood is warm.

VEGETABLE RISOTTO WITH TOFU

In this great-tasting high-protein meatless dish, the tofu, flavorless itself, takes on the tomato and cheese flavors. I've used broccoli as the vegetable, but you could substitute a 10-ounce package of frozen chopped spinach or 1 cup of grated carrots. Neither of these vegetables needs to be precooked. True risotto uses a short, round rice (Arborio) and has a creamy texture.

8 ounces firm tofu, drained
1 1/2 cups fresh broccoli
   florets
1 medium onion, chopped
1 clove garlic, minced
2 tablespoons vegetable oil
2/3 cup short-grain white
   rice
1/2 cup chicken stock plus
   1/2 cup more if necessary
One 16-ounce can tomato
   puree

1 teaspoon dried oregano
1/2 teaspoon basil
1 teaspoon sugar
1/2 teaspoon salt
1/2 teaspoon pepper
1/4 cup grated Parmesan
   cheese
1/2 cup grated Cheddar
   cheese, for topping

Preheat oven to 350°.

Cut the tofu into 1/2-inch pieces. Set aside.

In a small saucepan, steam the broccoli in about 1/2 inch of boiling water for about 5 minutes. Drain. Set aside.

In a large skillet, sauté the onion and garlic in the oil until translucent. Add the rice and stir until glazed; pour in the chicken stock and add the tomato puree. Bring to a boil and add the tofu, broccoli, oregano, basil, sugar, salt, and pepper. Lower heat and simmer for about 3 minutes.

Add the Parmesan cheese and pour the risotto into a greased 2-quart casserole. Bake uncovered for about 45 minutes, or until the rice, when tested is thoroughly cooked. Top with the Cheddar cheese and leave in the oven until melted, about 5 to 10 minutes. *Makes 4 or 5 servings.*

CREAMY RISOTTO WITH
APPLE AND CHEESE

This rice dish with its own sauce is perfect for meats that have no gravies, such as roast pork or chicken. Use a short-grained round rice. Many stores now carry rice labeled "for risotto."

1 1/2 cups short-grain white
  rice
4 tablespoons butter or
  margarine, divided
2 cups cooking apples,
  peeled and diced
5 cups chicken broth
1 tablespoon olive oil
3 tablespoons minced
  onion

1/2 cup dry white wine or
  7UP
2 cups mozzarella cheese,
  grated
1/3 cup grated Parmesan
  cheese
1/2 teaspoon nutmeg

Measure rice. Set aside.

In a large saucepan, heat 2 tablespoons of the butter over moderate heat. Add the apples and cook, stirring frequently, until the apples are tender. Remove to a bowl. Wipe the pan.

In another pan, bring the broth to a simmer. Keep hot.

In the first saucepan, heat the oil plus remaining butter. Add the onion and sauté it at medium heat until soft. Add the rice and stir for 1 minute, or until the grains are coated. Add the wine and stir until absorbed. Add the hot broth, 1/2 cup at a time, stirring frequently. Wait until each addition is almost absorbed before adding more. Reserve 1/4 cup.

Add the apples. When the rice is tender but not soft, about 18 minutes after starting, add the remaining 1/4 cup broth, the mozzarella and Parmesan cheeses, and the nutmeg. Stir vigorously. Serve the risotto when the cheese is fully melted and creamy. *Makes 6 servings.*

BEANS AND LENTILS

SWEDISH BROWN BEANS

This sweet and spicy bean casserole is classic at any Swedish smorgasbord, and is just as good for a hearty family supper. I prefer the large Swedish brown beans, but if you can't find them in your market, substitute navy or pinto beans and reduce the vinegar to 1/3 cup. As with most dried beans, these need to soak for an hour before cooking.

2 cups Swedish brown beans	1/4 cup molasses
1 cup chopped onion	1/2 cup cider vinegar
1 cup ketchup	1 teaspoon dry mustard
2 tablespoons Worcestershire sauce	3 tablespoons cornstarch
	4 slices Canadian bacon
1 cup dark brown sugar	1/4 to 1/2 cup water if needed for sauce

Wash and sort beans. Place them in a 5-quart pot or bowl. Pour enough boiling water over beans to cover by 2 inches. Cover and let stand for 1 hour. Drain. Cover beans with fresh water, bring to a boil, and cook at a simmer until beans are tender to bite. Since beans take various lengths of time to cook, start testing at 20 minutes. Drain and rinse once.

Preheat oven to 325°.

Place the beans in a 3-quart casserole. Add the onion.

In a saucepan, stir together the ketchup, Worcestershire sauce, sugar, molasses, vinegar, mustard, and cornstarch. Over medium heat, stir until cornstarch dissolves. Then mix the sauce in with the beans. Place the bacon on top, cover, and bake for 1 1/2 to 2 hours. *Makes 6 to 8 servings.*

HAWAIIAN PORK AND BEANS

New England missionaries carried their baked beans to Hawaii and there added this touch of Polynesia. Use for a cookout or take to a potluck dinner. For a quick canned-bean version, see Quick-bake Beans, below.

One 16-ounce package dry
  calico beans
1 pound ground pork
1 large onion, diced
2 tablespoons brown sugar
2¹/₂ teaspoons salt
1 heaping teaspoon dry
  mustard

¹/₂ teaspoon pepper
2 tablespoons molasses
1¹/₂ tablespoons GF
  vinegar
2 tablespoons lemon juice
One 8¹/₄-ounce can
  pineapple tidbits
¹/₂ cup ketchup

Wash and pick over the beans. Place in an 8-quart Dutch oven and add 8 cups of water. Bring to a boil over high heat and cook for 3 minutes. Cover and let stand for 1 hour. Drain the beans in a colander. Rinse with fresh water.

In the Dutch oven, cook the pork and onion over medium heat until pork is brown and onion is translucent. Stir to prevent burning. Return the beans to Dutch oven and add the sugar, salt, mustard, and pepper. Simmer for 1¹/₂ hours.

Stir in the molasses, vinegar, lemon juice, pineapple with its juice, and ketchup. At this point you may either bring to a boil, reduce heat to low, cover, and simmer for 15 minutes or more until the beans are tender, or you may put the Dutch oven in a 350° oven and bake, covered, for about 1 hour. The oven method results in the most flavorful beans. *Makes 10 to 12 servings.*

QUICK-BAKE METHOD: Use three 15-ounce cans of pinto beans with their liquid; add to the meat and onion browned in the Dutch oven. Stir in the rest of the ingredients. Bake, covered, for at least 45 minutes in a 350° oven. If the beans are too moist, remove lid for the final 15 minutes of baking.

BUTTER-BASTED LIMAS
WITH HAM

This super lima bean dish for a picnic, a party, or just plain family eating can be made ahead and reheated. The casserole is more flavorful when started with the dry beans, but if time is short, see the Quick-bake Method, below.

2 cups dried lima beans
1¹/₂-pound ham hock
One 5.5-ounce can V-8
  juice

Sauce

¹/₃ cup butter or
  margarine, melted

³/₄ cups sour cream or
  nondairy substitute
³/₄ cup brown sugar
3 tablespoons molasses
2 teaspoons dry mustard
Salt to taste

Soak beans overnight in cold water to cover by 1 inch. Drain.

Wash the ham hock and place it with the beans in a large kettle or Dutch oven. Add the V-8 juice and hot water to cover by about ¹/₂ inch. Boil for 1 hour. Drain.

Preheat oven to 350°.

Remove ham. Pick out meat and dice. Return the meat to the beans.

To make the sauce, combine the butter, sour cream, sugar, molasses, mustard, and salt.

Add the sauce to the beans. Pour them into a buttered 3-quart casserole or Dutch oven. Cover and bake for 30 minutes. Uncover and bake 30 more minutes. If too dry, return cover to casserole. *Makes 8 to 10 servings.*

QUICK-BAKE METHOD: Use four 15-ounce cans of drained butter beans. Cover with the sauce mix and add ¹/₂ cup cooked ham cut in bite-sized chunks. Bake as above.

LENTILS MARRAKESH
(with Chicken)

Spicy, hearty, and easy with all the flavor of old Morocco, this delicious but unusual main dish is a welcome change from rice or potatoes and meat. It requires long cooking, but you may use an electric Crock-Pot or simmer in a Dutch oven on top of the stove. Cook it the night before, if desired, for the flavor is even better when reheated. Serve with a green salad or sliced fruit for a full meal.

2 pounds chicken thighs, bone in
1 1/2 cups brown lentils
4 cups chicken broth or water
1 cup chopped onion
1 cup chopped celery (may use tops)
2 tablespoons ketchup
1 teaspoon ground turmeric
3/4 teaspoon ground cinnamon
2 to 3 tablespoons lemon juice
Salt and pepper to taste

Wash the chicken and lentils. Place them in a Crock-Pot or in a large Dutch oven. Add the chicken broth, onion, celery, ketchup, turmeric, and cinnamon. Cover and cook for 5 to 9 hours if in a CrockPot, or for 3 to 5 hours at a simmer if in a Dutch oven. Add more broth or water if necessary.

Before serving, remove the thighs, discard the skin and bones, and cut the meat into bite-sized pieces. Return to the pot and season with lemon juice and salt and pepper. *Makes 6 to 8 servings.*

PASTA

FRESH EGG PASTA

Making your own noodles or spaghetti may seem like a lot of trouble, but this pasta is so good you won't mind the bother. You don't need a pasta machine. With just one bowl and a little kneading, the dough is ready to be rolled out and cut into fettuccine, spaghetti, or lasagne noodles.

The pasta can be cooked and used immediately in any pasta recipe, or it can be frozen either cooked or uncooked. I have not found drying a successful way to preserve the pasta.

$^1/_2$ cup tapioca flour	$4^1/_2$ teaspoons xanthan
$^1/_2$ cup cornstarch	gum
3 tablespoons potato	3 large eggs (see Note)
starch flour	$1^1/_2$ tablespoons vegetable
$^3/_4$ teaspoon salt	oil

In a medium bowl, combine flours, salt, and xanthan gum.

Beat the eggs lightly and add the oil. Pour the egg-oil liquid into the flour mixture and stir. This will feel much like pastry dough. Work the dough into a firm ball. Knead for 1 or 2 minutes.

Making pasta shapes without a pasta machine: Place the ball of dough on a potato starch–floured (rice flour turns noodles gray) breadboard and roll as *thin as possible*. This dough is tough and, when almost transparent, will still handle well. (One pasta book suggests you should see the board through the dough.) Cut into desired shape. For fettuccine and spaghetti, slice very thin strips. For a noodle casserole, make slightly wider noodles. If using for lasagne, cut into $1^1/_2$-by-4-inch rectangles.

Making pasta shapes with a machine: If you have the pasta attachment for a KitchenAid mixer, follow machine directions and drop the walnut-sized balls of dough into the top. If you have one of the pasta-cutting machines like Atlas, you might need to roll the dough slightly to get a sheet started for the cutters. Just follow the directions on your machine for the finished product. *Serves 4 for spaghetti, fettuccine, etc. or 6 to 8 in a noodle casserole.*

For chow mein noodles: Cut pasta as for spaghetti. Then cut these strips into 1-by-1¹/₂-inch lengths. Drop, uncooked, into hot oil and cook for a few seconds. Remove from oil and drain on paper towels. Use immediately in a casserole or one of the oriental dishes, or freeze for later. *Makes about 8 cups chow mein noodles.*

To cook pasta: Cook in salted boiling water, to which 1 tablespoon of oil has been added, for about 10 to 12 minutes depending on the thickness and size of your pieces. You will have to test for doneness. Drain and rinse well.

NOTE: If you are watching your cholesterol, egg whites turn out an excellent noodle. Add one or two more whites than the number of whole eggs called for in the recipe.

FETTUCCINE WITH SHRIMP AND SCALLOPS

A simple, flavorful, quick-cooking seafood sauce for pasta. Use either Fresh Egg Pasta or purchased GF fettuccine.

1 batch Fresh Egg Pasta (page 228) or 12 ounces GF fettuccine

4 tablespoons vegetable or olive oil, divided

¹/₂ pound bay scallops

¹/₂ pound uncooked shrimp

¹/₂ cup onion, chopped

2 cloves garlic, minced

1 tablespoon sweet rice flour

¹/₂ teaspoon coriander

3 tablespoons sherry

1 cup rich milk or nondairy liquid

Salt and pepper to taste

2 tablespoons fresh parsley, chopped

Cook the pasta in salted boiling water with 1 tablespoon of the oil until tender. Drain.

Meanwhile, wash the scallops. Wash, peel, and devein the shrimp. Put aside.

In a large, heavy skillet, heat the remaining 3 tablespoons oil over medium high heat. Add the onion and garlic and sauté until onion is clear. Stir in the flour and coriander. Cook for about 1/2 minute. Add the sherry and milk and bring to a boil, stirring constantly. Add the shrimp and scallops and simmer for about 5 minutes, or until shrimp are cooked through. Stir occasionally. Season with salt and pepper.

Just before serving, stir in the parsley. Arrange fettuccine on plates and spoon on the sauce. *Makes 4 generous servings.*

TOUCH-OF-IRISH CASSEROLE

This noodle dish with great flavor can be made ahead to pull from the refrigerator and bake at the last minute. If prepared early, cool the sauce before adding to the casserole. For the lactose intolerant, substitute 1/2 pound of tofu in 1/2-inch squares for the cheese.

3/4 batch Fresh Egg Pasta
  noodles (page 228) or 8
  ounces GF pasta
1 1/2 cups cooked corned
  beef, diced, or one 12-
  ounce can corned beef
1/4 pound (1 cup) grated
  Swiss cheese
4 green onions, sliced thin
1/2 cup slivered almonds,
  for topping (optional)

Sauce

2 tablespoons butter or
  margarine
2 tablespoons sweet rice
  flour
1 cup chicken broth
1 cup rich milk or
  nondairy liquid
Salt and pepper to taste

Cook the pasta in salted boiling water until tender. Drain and combine in a greased 2-quart casserole with the corned beef, cheese, and green onions.

Preheat oven to 350°.

Sauce: In a medium saucepan, melt the butter; add the flour and stir in the chicken broth; cook slightly. Add the milk and cook, stirring constantly, until thickened. Season with salt and pepper.

Pour the hot sauce over the ingredients in the casserole and toss gently until well mixed. Add the almonds, if desired. Bake for 45 minutes. *Makes 6 servings.*

SAVORY HAM CASSEROLE

A tasty pasta casserole that uses leftover ham and celery in a light cheese sauce. Serve with a tossed salad or fruit for a full meal. See below for a chicken variation.

1 to 1¹/₂ cups cooked ham
1¹/₂ cups Fresh Egg Pasta
  (page 228) or GF
  noodles
¹/₂ cup chopped celery
¹/₄ cup crushed potato
  chips or sliced almonds,
  for topping

Sauce

3 tablespoons butter or
  margarine

3 tablespoons rice flour
¹/₂ teaspoon salt
1¹/₂ cups milk or nondairy
  liquid
¹/₂ cup grated Cheddar
  cheese
3 green onions, sliced thin
¹/₄ cup almonds or
  cashews, chopped

Dice the ham. Cook the pasta in salted water with a few drops of vegetable oil until tender. Drain.

Preheat oven to 375°.

Sauce: in a 2-quart saucepan, melt the butter, stir in the flour and salt, then slowly add the milk. Cook to thicken, stirring constantly. Melt in the cheese. Remove from heat and add onions and almonds along with the noodles, ham, and celery. Mix well and pour into a 2¹/₂-quart greased baking dish. Top with the potato chips. Bake for 30 to 35 minutes. *Makes 4 servings.*

CHICKEN-BROCCOLI SUPREME: Replace the ham with chicken and the celery with 1 cup of uncooked broccoli steamed for about 3 minutes.

LAMB KASHA WITH PINE NUTS

In Lebanon this tasty main dish casserole would be made with cracked wheat, but I've substituted kasha (roasted buckwheat kernels). Buckwheat is of the rhubarb family and is not considered to contain gluten (see page 15). This casserole is well worth the time it takes to put together.

1 tablespoon vegetable oil	1/8 teaspoon cinnamon
1 1/2 pounds ground lamb	1 cup kasha
2/3 cup minced onion	1 egg, beaten slightly
1/2 cup pine nuts	2 cups chicken broth
1 1/2 teaspoons salt	2 tablespoons butter or
1/2 teaspoon pepper	margarine

Preheat oven to 350°.

In a large frying pan, heat the oil. Add the lamb and onion and cook until no pink shows on the meat, stirring frequently. Add the pine nuts, 1/2 teaspoon of the salt, 1/4 teaspoon of the pepper, and the cinnamon. Remove from heat and pour the mixture into a bowl. Wipe the pan.

In a small bowl, combine the kasha with the egg. In a small saucepan, bring the broth, the remaining 1 teaspoon salt and 1/4 teaspoon pepper, and the butter to a boil.

Return the frying pan to the heat and pour in the egg-coated kasha. Stir the kasha until each kernel is dry and separate, about 2 to 4 minutes. Pour on the hot broth, cover, reduce heat to low, and cook for about 10 minutes.

Combine meat and cooked kasha and pour into a buttered 1 1/2-quart casserole. Bake for 1 hour. *Makes 6 servings.*

VEGETABLES

POTATOES

Baked Chips
Princess Potatoes
Colcannon
Potato Patties with Apple
 and Cheese
Potato Baskets

VEGETABLE CASSEROLES

Ratatouille
Broccoli-Cheese Almondine
Cauliflower Casserole
Vegetable and Cheese Strata
Corn Soufflé
Spaghetti Squash Casserole
Vegetable Parmigiana
Old-fashioned Creamed
 Cabbage

TEMPURA

Tempura Batter for
 Vegetables
Dipping Sauce for
 Tempura

SALADS

Soufflé Salad
Two-Tone Molded Vegetable
 Salad

PICKLES

Sweet Chunk Pickles
Icicle Pickles

SAUCE

Tomato Sauce

We can have vegetables steamed, boiled, stir-fried, or baked. Usually I serve them one of these ways. But sometimes, for a change, it's exciting to vary their tastes by blending them in casseroles or salads or even turning them into pickles.

This short section includes my testers' favorite casseroles using vegetables as a base, a recipe for GF tempura batter, plus two beautiful molded vegetable salads wonderful for parties or potlucks—they feed a crowd and have proved popular every time I've served them. I've also included several ways, some of them quite different, to use potatoes.

Because most pickles on the grocery shelves contain distilled vinegar, I've included two pickle recipes. Some GF pickles are available at health food stores, but since I've started making my own during cucumber season, I prefer them to any "store-boughten" ones.

POTATOES

BAKED CHIPS

A baked version of the English chip, or our French fry, these are lower in cholesterol and much easier to digest. You can eat them for snacks as well as an accompaniment to your fish or shrimp.

> 4 fist-sized potatoes, washed and well scrubbed,
>   not peeled
> 2 tablespoons mayonnaise
> 1 tablespoon milk or nondairy liquid
> Lemon pepper

Preheat oven to 375°.

Cut the potatoes lengthwise into quarters and each quarter into 3 wedges (yielding 12 wedges per potato). Place the wedges on a well-greased cookie sheet.

Thin the mayonnaise with the milk and brush on the potato wedges. Sprinkle the pieces liberally with lemon pepper. Bake for 50 minutes, or until golden brown and tender. Remove from the cookie sheet while still hot. *Makes 2 or 3 servings.*

PRINCESS POTATOES

When a guest asks for a recipe, a hostess knows she has a hit. This casserole prompted two such requests the first time I served it. Serve these make-ahead potatoes with meats that have no gravies, such as ham, Turkey Loaf (page 308), or your favorite barbecued specialty.

6 fist-sized new potatoes
1 cup sour cream or
    nondairy substitute
$1/2$ cup milk or nondairy
    liquid
3 eggs, slightly beaten
$1/2$ cup chopped onion

1 cup grated Monterey
    Jack cheese
$3/4$ teaspoon salt
$1/2$ teaspoon pepper
$1/2$ cup grated Cheddar
    cheese

Preheat oven to 350°.

Boil the potatoes until almost cooked, about 15 minutes. Cool. Then peel and grate into a large mixing bowl.

Add the sour cream, milk, eggs, onion, Monterey Jack cheese, salt, and pepper. Mix well and pour into a buttered 9″ × 13″ casserole or baking dish. (If making ahead, cover with plastic wrap and refrigerate.)

Bake for 30 minutes. Then remove from oven to sprinkle the Cheddar cheese on top. Return to oven for 10 to 15 minutes longer to let the cheese melt. *Makes 8 servings.*

COLCANNON

Serve this Irish potato and cabbage combination with corned beef if you wish, but it goes equally well with anything from roast beef to meat loaf, pork roast to chops. The wonderful flavor needs no gravy.

6 medium boiling potatoes	1/4 cup water
1/3 cup rich milk	3 cups shredded green
3 tablespoons margarine or	cabbage (1/2 large head)
butter, plus margarine or	2 leeks or 6 green onions,
butter for topping	chopped
1 slice bacon, diced, or 1	Salt to taste
tablespoon vegetable oil	Pepper to taste

Peel the potatoes and cook in salted water (1 cup water to 1 teaspoon salt). When cooked, drain and mash with the milk and margarine until fluffy.

Meanwhile, in a large saucepan, fry the bacon. Remove the bits but save the grease (or use only the vegetable oil). Add the water, shredded cabbage, leeks, and salt. Cover and simmer until tender, 5 to 10 minutes. Drain thoroughly.

Combine the cabbage with the whipped potatoes and beat again. Season with salt and pepper, dot with margarine, and serve immediately. *Makes 6 servings.*

POTATO PATTIES WITH
APPLE AND CHEESE

A tasty old German way with potatoes that originally called for grating the ingredients. With a food processor, you can save a lot of time (and some scraped knuckles). Serve with turkey, meat loaf, ham, or other meats that don't have a gravy.

4 fist-sized potatoes,
  cooked in their skins
2 crisp cooking apples,
  peeled and cored
1 medium onion, cubed
4 tablespoons grated Swiss
  cheese

$^1/_2$ teaspoon tarragon
$^1/_2$ teaspoon nutmeg
$^1/_4$ teaspoon pepper
Salt to taste
1 tablespoon vegetable oil,
  for frying

Peel the potatoes. Put in a food processor along with the apples and onion. Process until just chopped. (Or you may grate each separately.) Place the chopped mixture in a mixing bowl. Add the cheese, tarragon, nutmeg, pepper, and salt. Mix thoroughly. Let stand for 10 to 30 minutes for flavors to meld.

Form 3-inch patties and fry in oil on both sides to sear, then lower heat to medium and cook through, about 10 minutes. *Makes 6 to 8 servings.*

POTATO BASKETS

Potatoes, hollowed out and baked as baskets, are a flavorful and healthy change from pastry shells. I've filled them with Chicken à la King (page 269) or creamed salmon or tuna, or have smothered them with grated cheese, bacon bits, and chopped green onions, then stuck them under the broiler for a few minutes, until the cheese melted.

   6 baking potatoes
   1¹/₂ tablespoons mayonnaise diluted to brushing
      consistency with milk or nondairy liquid
   Lemon pepper or salt and pepper

Preheat oven to 375°.

Thoroughly scrub the potatoes. Cut a lengthwise slice off the top of each so they resemble baskets. Take a thin slice off each bottom to make a flat base.

With a melon baller, scoop out the inside of each potato, leaving a ¹/₄-inch shell. Brush the inside with the diluted mayonnaise and season with the lemon pepper. Place on a greased baking sheet and bake for 35 to 40 minutes.

Fill and serve while still hot or, if made ahead, reheat and then fill. *Makes 6 servings.*

VEGETABLE CASSEROLES

RATATOUILLE

This casserole of mixed vegetables is an easy fix-ahead dish for the cook, and it's even tastier if made hours before serving. Once baked, serve at room temperature or reheat, as desired. Ratatouille is excellent as a barbecue or potluck side dish. The suggested vegetables are basic, but you may add to them any or all of the following: sliced carrots, sliced yellow squash, or sliced small, delicate zucchini (large ones contain too much moisture). Experiment with different colored vegetables for an exciting look to your casserole.

1 medium eggplant, cubed
1 large onion, sliced or
   chopped
2 to 3 cloves garlic,
   minced
2 large tomatoes, peeled,
   seeded, and chopped, or
   one 16-ounce can whole
   tomatoes, drained and
   chopped
$^1/_2$ medium red or green
   bell pepper, seeded and
   chopped

$^1/_2$ cup minced fresh
   parsley
$^1/_2$ teaspoon oregano or
   marjoram
1 to $1^1/_2$ teaspoons salt,
   to taste
$^1/_3$ cup olive oil
$^1/_4$ teaspoon thyme
   (optional)

Preheat oven to 300° or 325°.

Place all ingredients in a $2^1/_2$-quart casserole. Fill to the top; the vegetables will cook down considerably. Bake for 1 hour in a 325° oven $1^1/_2$ hours or at 300° for 2 hours. *Makes 6 to 8 servings.*

BROCCOLI-CHEESE ALMONDINE

A great party dish but easy enough for any family dinner, this almondine is so good you won't have any leftovers. This recipe may easily be doubled; use a 2-quart casserole. You will not need to double the almonds.

2 to 3 cups broccoli florets and stems	2 tablespoons rice flour
2 tablespoons margarine	1 cup milk or nondairy liquid
2 tablespoons chopped onions	1 cup Cheddar cheese, grated
1/2 teaspoon salt	1 cup sliced almonds

Preheat oven to 350°.

Cook the broccoli until barely tender. Drain and place it in a buttered 1 1/2-quart casserole.

In a medium saucepan, melt the margarine and sauté the onion until clear. Stir in the salt and flour. Add the milk slowly, stirring continually. Turn heat to medium and cook until sauce has thickened. Add the cheese and stir until cheese melts. Spoon the cheese sauce over the broccoli. Top with the almonds. Bake for 30 minutes. *Makes 3 or 4 servings.*

CAULIFLOWER CASSEROLE

Cauliflower dressed up with a wonderful sauce is a make-ahead company dish easy enough for the family.

1 head cauliflower

Sauce

1½ tablespoons butter or
   margarine
3 tablespoons rice flour
¾ cup chicken stock
½ cup milk or nondairy
   liquid

1 green onion, sliced thin
¼ teaspoon salt or to taste
Pepper to taste
½ cup mayonnaise
1 tablespoon lemon juice
½ cup grated Cheddar
   cheese
¼ cup sliced almonds, for
   garnish

Preheat oven to 350°.

Wash the cauliflower and break it into florets. Precook by steaming for 5 minutes or place in a covered casserole and microwave on high for 5 minutes. Place in buttered 2-quart casserole.

Sauce: In a saucepan, melt the butter. Add the flour and stir. Slowly add the chicken stock, stirring constantly to prevent lumping. Add the milk and cook, stirring, until mixture comes to a boil. Add the onion, salt, and pepper, and cook for 1 minute more. Remove from heat.

Stir in the mayonnaise, lemon juice, and cheese. Pour the sauce over the cauliflower and sprinkle on the almonds. Bake for 30 to 40 minutes. *Makes 4 or 5 servings.*

VEGETABLE AND
CHEESE STRATA

Strata means layers *in Italian, and that is just how this simple but colorful casserole is prepared. You may use any combination of fresh vegetables and cheeses you wish as long as the combination is pleasing to the eye and palate. Try broccoli and yellow bell pepper; mushrooms, green onions, and carrots; califlower and red or green peppers. Avoid watery vegetables such as eggplant and large zucchini.*

This makes a full meal with a simple fruit salad, or it can accompany fish, ham, or chicken.

1 tablespoon butter or margarine
1 cup (¹/₂ pound) fresh asparagus, in 1-inch pieces
1 cup carrots, diced
¹/₄ cup onion, chopped
3 cups GF bread in ¹/₂-inch cubes

1¹/₃ cups Monterey Jack or Swiss cheese, shredded
1¹/₃ cups milk or nondairy liquid
3 eggs, beaten
¹/₂ teaspoon salt
¹/₄ teaspoon paprika

In a large frying pan, heat the butter and stir in the asparagus and carrots. Cook over medium-high heat for 2 minutes. Add the onion and cook until the vegetables are crisp tender. (Cover, if desired, for more moistness.) Put aside to cool.

Into a greased 2-quart casserole place half the bread cubes. Top with half the vegetable mixture and half the cheese, Repeat layers.

Combine the milk, eggs, salt, and paprika. Pour over the casserole. Cover and refrigerate for several hours.

Preheat oven to 350°. Bake covered for approximately 40 minutes; remove the cover and cook another 10 minutes, or until the center is set and the top is browned. *Makes 6 servings.*

CORN SOUFFLÉ

This never-fail vegetable soufflé is a tasty way of stretching one can of corn for a meatless dish. As a main dish, serve with a salad; as a side dish, pair with ham, chicken, or fish. This can be prepared ahead and baked as guests gather.

One 17-ounce can whole kernel corn
$3/4$ cup (approximately) milk or nondairy liquid
$1/4$ cup margarine or butter
$1/3$ cup cornmeal
3 eggs, separated

$1/2$ teaspoon baking powder
$1/4$ teaspoon salt
Dash cayenne pepper
1 to 3 tablespoons bell pepper (as desired), minced
3 to 4 sliced green onions

Preheat oven to 375°.

Drain the corn, saving the liquid. Add the milk to the liquid to measure $1^1/2$ cups. In a saucepan combine the milk mixture and margarine, and bring to a boil. Slowly stir in the cornmeal. Bring back to a boil and cook for 3 minutes, stirring constantly. Remove from heat.

Beat the egg whites until stiff.

To the egg yolks, add the baking powder, salt, cayenne pepper, bell pepper, onions, and corn. Stir the corn mixture into the cooked meal. Fold in the egg whites. Pour into a buttered $1^1/2$-quart casserole.

Bake for 30 minutes, or until lightly browned and set. *Makes 4 servings as a main dish; 6 to 8 servings as a side dish.*

SPAGHETTI SQUASH CASSEROLE

A great casserole! Don't pass up this dish even if you've don't like spaghetti squash and tomato sauce. Here the mild turkey ham and Swiss cheese complement the flavor of this unique vegetable.

One 2-pound spaghetti
  squash
4 tablespoons butter or
  margarine
2 cups cooked turkey ham,
  diced
1 cup sliced mushrooms,
  fresh or canned
1 medium onion, diced
3 tablespoons rice flour
1 cup milk or nondairy
  liquid

1 cup chicken broth
1 1/2 cups grated Swiss
  cheese
1 1/2 teaspoons prepared
  mustard
1/2 teaspoon salt
Dash pepper
1/3 cup grated Cheddar
  cheese (optional)
1/2 cup slivered almonds
  (optional)

Preheat oven to 350°.

Cook the squash by cutting in half lengthwise and baking, cut side down, in a 9″ × 13″ baking pan or casserole for about 30 minutes, or until the meat feels tender. Cool and remove seeds and inside pith. Remove the spaghetti-like strands gently with a fork and place in a large mixing bowl (there should be about 5 cups).

In a large skillet, melt the butter. Sauté the ham and mushrooms briefly. Add the mixture to the squash.

In the same skillet, sauté the onion until clear. Add the flour and pour in the combined milk and chicken broth, stirring until smooth and thickened. Add 3/4 cup of the Swiss cheese, the mustard, salt, and pepper, and stir until the cheese is melted. Pour this into the bowl of spaghetti squash mixture. Tumble gently until mixed and place in a buttered 9″ × 13″ pan or casserole. Bake for 25 minutes. Top with the remaining Swiss cheese, the Cheddar, if used, and the almonds, if used. Return to the oven for another 5 to 7 minutes. *Makes 6 servings.*

VEGETABLE PARMIGIANA

An unusual dish of eggplant or yellow squash and zucchini. Serve this when you crave a high-protein meatless entrée. Add a green salad and one of the breads (pages 33 to 91) and you have a full meal. These individual serving dishes can be prepared ahead to be cooked at dinnertime (allow a little more baking time if the casseroles have been refrigerated).

1 medium eggplant or 2 cups sliced yellow squash	1/2 cup grated mozzarella cheese
2 cups sliced zucchini	One 14-ounce jar GF spaghetti sauce
Salt to taste	1/4 cup grated Parmesan cheese
1 cup ricotta cheese	

Preheat oven to 350°F.

Peel the eggplant and cut into 1/2-inch-thick slices; cut slices in half. Wash and bias-slice the zucchini. (If using yellow squash, treat as zucchini.) Cook the vegetables in boiling salted water for about 4 minutes.

Divide the cooked vegetables into 4 au gratin dishes or individual casseroles. Top each with 1/4 cup of the ricotta cheese and 2 tablespoons of the mozzarella. Divide the spaghetti sauce equally over the dishes. Top with the remaining mozzarella and the Parmesan. Bake, uncovered, for 25 to 30 minutes, or until heated through and bubbly. *Makes 4 servings.*

OLD-FASHIONED
CREAMED CABBAGE

Cabbage in a casserole may sound old-fashioned when we can serve fresh (imported and expensive) summer vegetables all winter, but try this once and you'll understand why it's still popular in many countries. This is a hearty dish, so pair it with some leftover roast, ham, or chicken. Serve fruit for dessert to help lower the calories. For variety, add one grated apple to the casserole before baking.

1 medium-size head green cabbage
2 eggs, beaten
1 tablespoon butter or margarine, melted
3/4 teaspoon salt
1/4 teaspoon pepper
1/4 cup cream or nondairy liquid, undiluted
1/2 cup grated Cheddar cheese, for topping (optional)

Preheat oven to 400°.

Wash, core, and shred the cabbage. Cook until tender. Drain. In a large bowl, combine the cabbage with the rest of the ingredients except the Cheddar cheese and then pour them into a buttered 3-quart casserole or baking dish.

Bake for about 15 minutes. Add the cheese topping, if desired, and return to oven for another 5 to 7 minutes. *Makes 6 to 8 servings.*

TEMPURA

TEMPURA BATTER FOR
VEGETABLES

The unusual combination of flavors plus the delicate texture make this batter for deep-frying vegetables a winner, even for those who can have gluten. Use for Japanese-style onion rings, zucchini strips, thin potato slices, broccoli bits, green beans, mushrooms, or any vegetable you choose. To be authentically Japanese, serve with a dipping sauce.

1 egg, beaten
1/4 cup cornstarch
1/2 cup rice flour (sweet rice is best)
1/4 teaspoon xanthan gum
1 teaspoon seasoning salt
Salt to taste (if necessary)

1/2 teaspoon baking powder
1 cup Fresca, 7UP, or Sprite
3 cups vegetable oil, for deep frying
2 cups washed and cut-up vegetables

In a medium bowl, beat the egg.

Mix together the cornstarch, rice flour, xanthan gum, seasoning salt, salt, and baking powder. Stir the dry mix into the egg alternately with the Fresca.

Heat the oil in an automatic frying kettle or frying pan to 375°. Dip the vegetables into the batter, then gently drop them into the hot oil, cooking only a few pieces at a time. Turn once as they brown. Remove and drain on paper toweling. Serve while hot with or without dipping sauce, page 250. *Makes 4 servings.*

DIPPING SAUCE

This may be made ahead and cooled before preparing the tempura. One tester says she cooked the radish and ginger with the sauce. Excellent.

1/4 cup GF soy sauce
1/4 cup dry sherry
1 cup chicken stock
Dash salt or to taste

1 daikon radish, grated
1 finger (2 tablespoons)
  fresh gingerroot, grated

In a small saucepan, place the soy sauce, sherry, chicken stock, and salt. Bring to a boil over medium heat. Remove and let cool. When ready to serve, pour into separate small bowls for each diner.

Place bowls of the radish and the ginger on the table and let each diner season the sauce to taste by adding the grated pieces. *Makes 6 servings.*

SALADS

SOUFFLÉ SALAD

Serve this crunchy, cool-looking molded vegetable salad with a summer meal. For a firmer mold, add 1/2 teaspoon plain gelatin.

One 6-ounce package
  lemon gelatin
2 cups hot water
1 cup cold water
1 cup mayonnaise
4 tablespoons vinegar
1 teaspoon salt
3 cups shredded green
  cabbage

1 cup diced celery
1 cup sliced radishes
1/4 cup minced onion
1/4 cup green bell pepper,
  minced
Lettuce, for serving
Extra radishes, for garnish

In a large bowl, dissolve the gelatin in the 2 cups hot water.

Mix together the 1 cup cold water, the mayonnaise, vinegar, and salt. Stir into the gelatin. Refrigerate until not quite jelled.

Remove from the refrigerator and whip with eggbeater. Stir in the cabbage, celery, radishes, onions, and bell pepper. Pour into an oiled 2-quart mold and refrigerate from 3 hours to overnight. Unmold onto a lettuce-lined serving plate and garnish with radish roses. *Makes 12 servings.*

TWO-TONE MOLDED VEGETABLE SALAD

A beautiful vegetable salad that will fool everyone into thinking you've added tuna fish or poultry to the filling. A crowd pleaser at parties and potlucks. Add 1/2 teaspoon extra plain gelatin for a slightly firmer salad, if desired.

One 16-ounce can V-8 juice
One 8-ounce can tomato sauce
2 tablespoons apple cider vinegar
One 6-ounce package lemon gelatin
4 tablespoons minced green bell pepper

1 cup diced celery
2 cups grated green cabbage
2 cups cottage cheese
1/2 cup mayonnaise
Lettuce, for serving (optional)
Mayonnaise and paprika, for garnish (optional)

In a saucepan, bring to a boil the V-8 juice and tomato sauce.

Add the vinegar and pour the tomato mixture over the gelatin in a large mixing bowl. Pour one-fourth of the mixture into a 2-quart ring mold or a 9″ × 12″ pan. Refrigerate until set, about 25 minutes. Meanwhile, prepare the vegetables.

Blend together the cottage cheese and mayonnaise. Stir into the liquid gelatin. Add the vegetables. Pour this over the firm first layer in pan or mold. Refrigerate for at least 4 hours (overnight is better).

Serve from the pan by cutting into squares and turning the aspic side up on individual plates, or unmold entire salad onto a large platter garnished with lettuce. Top each serving with a dab of mayonnaise and a sprinkle of paprika, if desired. *Makes 12 servings.*

PICKLES

SWEET CHUNK PICKLES

Since many of the pickles on the market contain distilled vinegar, you might want to put up your own during cucumber season. These are easy to make and wonderfully good. Most sweet pickles take almost two weeks, but these can be soaked in brine overnight and put into the spiced vinegar the next day.

8 to 10 cups 2- to 3-inch cucumbers, cut into 1-inch chunks	3 tablespoons whole mixed pickling spices
2 quarts cold water	1 teaspoon whole cloves
$^2/_3$ cup salt	One 3-inch cinnamon stick, broken
6 cups apple cider vinegar	$^1/_2$ teaspoon alum (optional; see Note)
4 cups sugar	

Place the cucumbers in a large glass bowl or crock.

In a medium bowl, add a small amount of the cold water to the salt, let that dissolve, then add the rest. Cover the cucumbers with this brine. Let set 24 hours.

In a saucepan mix the vinegar, sugar, pickling spices, cloves, cinnamon, and alum, if used. Bring to the boiling point.

Drain off the brine and immediately pour boiling water over to cover the chunks. Drain in a colander and immediately pack the chunks tightly in hot sterilized jars. Cover at once with the vinegar mixture.

Seal jars with fresh caps and rings and process in a boiling water bath for 10 minutes.

Makes 5 to 6 pints.

NOTE: Alum is not an essential ingredient, but it will keep the pickles crisp and help retain the color.

ICICLE PICKLES

These crisp, sweet pickles are so good you won't mind the two weeks' time and the several processes involved in making them. By using cider vinegar, you can be sure they are gluten free. Since pickles keep well, you won't have to make them up every year unless, like me, you enjoy chopping them into salad dressings and all sandwich fillings. Use these for the Haitian Chicken (page 300).

3 quarts small pickling cucumbers, cut lengthwise in quarters	1 1/2 tablespoons mixed pickling spices
3/4 cup salt	5 cups sugar
1 1/2 quarts water	5 cups apple cider vinegar

Place the cucumber strips in a stone jar or large glass container.

Add the salt to the water and bring to boiling. Pour the brine over the cucumbers. Cover with a fitted plate or saucer and top with a weight (a sealed jar of water can replace Grandma's washed stone). Let stand one week.

After a week, drain, discarding the brine. Rinse the cucumbers thoroughly and cover with boiling water. Cover and let stand 24 hours.

Drain. Cover with boiling water; cover and let stand 24 hours. Drain.

Tie the spices in a cheesecloth bag. In a saucepan, bring to a boil the spices, sugar, and vinegar. Pour the mixture over the cucumbers. Cover and let stand 24 hours.

Drain the syrup; bring it to a boil again and then pour it over cucumbers. Repeat this step 3 more times.

The next day, drain the cucumbers, reserving the syrup; pack pickles into sterile pint canning jars, leaving one-quarter inch headspace. Discard the spice bag. Reheat the syrup to boiling and pour it over the pickles, leaving one-quarter inch headspace. Adjust fresh caps and rings. Process the jars in a boiling water bath for 10 minutes. *Makes about 6 pints.*

SAUCE

TOMATO SAUCE

A basic sauce to accompany many dishes. Serve it over Moussaka (page 274) or Russian Cabbage Rolls (page 276) or use it to spice up grits or noodles. Add more sugar or different spices to suit your tastes. Even the acidity of the tomatoes will vary the flavor.

1 tablespoon olive oil
2/3 cup minced onion
1 clove garlic, minced
2 cups ripe tomatoes, chopped (see Note)
1/2 cup water
1 1/2 teaspoons salt
1 teaspoon dried basil
1/2 teaspoon oregano

1/4 teaspoon pepper
1 crushed bay leaf
1 teaspoon sugar, or to taste
One 6-ounce can tomato paste
1/4 cup Burgundy (optional)

In a large saucepan, heat the oil, add the onion and garlic, and sauté over medium heat until onion is translucent. Add the tomatoes, water, salt, basil, oregano, pepper, bay leaf, and sugar. Bring to a boil, stirring constantly, then reduce heat to a simmer. Cook for 30 minutes, then add the tomato paste and Burgundy, if you are using it. If you don't use the wine, it may be necessary to thin with a bit more water to achieve the desired consistency. Leave the sauce on very low heat for at least another half hour for the flavors to meld. *Makes about 1 quart sauce.*

NOTE: You may substitute one 14^1/$_2$-ounce can whole tomatoes. Chop them and use the liquid, but eliminate the ^{1}/$_2$ cup of water from the recipe.

LUNCHEON AND SUPPER DISHES

EGG-BASED DISHES

Quiche with a Hash Brown
   Crust
Crab or Lobster Quiche
Egg Fu Yung

SANDWICHES

Crab-Cheese Melt
Gyros Sandwich
Bette's Special Filled Buns

CASSEROLES

Jeanne's Incredible Turkey
   Casserole

Austrian Cheese Puff
Sausage and Cheese Strata

CREAMED DISH

Chicken à la King

LUNCHEON SALAD

Taco Salad

Stuck for a quick dish for supper? Or do you want something elegant for that luncheon coming up? This section contains a wide variety of dishes for which you'll never have to apologize for being gluten free; these are all taste approved by testers and their families.

I did not include any pizzas in this book since I concentrated on them in *The Gluten-free Gourmet*, but if you need a pizza crust, make a recipe of the Crumpets (page 75) or Australian Toaster Buns (page 76) and, instead of forming six circles, spread all the batter in a twelve-inch circle on a greased and rice-floured pizza tin or cookie sheet, leaving a thicker crust around the outside edges to keep the sauce and fillings from spilling over. Let the dough rise for about 10 minutes before adding the toppings and then bake immediately in a 375° oven for 25 to 30 minutes.

EGG-BASED DISHES

QUICHE WITH A HASH BROWN CRUST

A tasty luncheon quiche using your choice of meats and cheeses. The recipe was given to me by a celiac acquaintance and proved so good, I've made it up several ways. If you can find a commercial frozen variety of hash brown potatoes that you know aren't dusted with wheat flour, you can substitute them for potatoes you grate yourself.

Crust

3 cups grated raw potatoes
(5 to 6 medium
potatoes)
1/3 cup butter or
margarine, melted

Filling

1/2 cup cooked sausage or
1/2 cup cooked ham,
diced, or 6 slices bacon,
fried, drained, and
crumbled

5 eggs
1/4 cup diced onion
1/2 cup grated Cheddar
cheese
1/4 cup grated Swiss or
Monterey Jack cheese
1 teaspoon dried basil
1 teaspoon chopped chives
Salt and pepper to taste
3/4 cup rich milk or
nondairy liquid

Preheat oven to 425°.

Crust: Coat a large pie plate with vegetable spray. Press in the potatoes to an even half-inch depth on bottom and up sides. Pour the butter evenly over the potatoes. Bake for 30 minutes.

Filling: Prepare your choice of meats and set aside. In a large mixing bowl, beat the eggs; add the onion, cheeses, basil, chives, and salt and pepper. Stir in the milk and meat. Pour gently over the partially baked crust and return to the oven with the temperature lowered to 350°. Bake for 40 to 45 minutes, or until the center is set and a knife inserted comes out clean. Serve immediately. *Makes 4 to 6 servings.*

CRAB OR LOBSTER QUICHE

The easy crust and the seafood taste make this quiche one of my favorites. You may substitute gluten-free sirimi for the lobster or crab. The results are still excellent.

Crust

3/4 cup GF bread crumbs
3/4 cup crushed potato
  chips
Dash paprika
1/3 cup grated Parmesan
  cheese
4 tablespoons butter or
  margarine, melted

Filling

2 tablespoons rice flour
1/2 teaspoon salt

2 eggs, beaten
1/2 cup mayonnaise
1/2 cup rich milk or
  nondairy liquid,
  undiluted
2 cups cooked lobster,
  cubed, or crabmeat
1 cup grated Swiss cheese
1/4 cup sliced green onion

Preheat oven to 350°.

Crust: In a plastic bag, combine the bread crumbs, potato chips, paprika, and Parmesan cheese. Pour in the melted butter and blend. Pat into a deep 9″ pie pan.

Filling: Blend together the flour, salt, eggs, mayonnaise, and milk. Add the lobster, Swiss cheese, and onion. Pour into the pie shell. Bake for 45 minutes, or until a knife inserted in the center comes out clean. *Makes 6 servings.*

EGG FU YUNG

This flavorful and easy Chinese omelette uses fresh vegetables with left-over pork or chicken. Or substitute cooked crab or shrimp for an entirely different taste. My favorite, the shrimp, tastes like egg roll. You may add other vegetables such as finely slivered zucchini, diced water chestnuts, or chopped bamboo shoots. Serve Ginger-Orange Rolls (page 76) and fruit or salad for a wonderful luncheon or supper.

1/2 cup cooked chicken, pork, shrimp, or crab	1 teaspoon salt
1/2 cup chopped onion	2 teaspoons GF soy sauce
1/2 cup finely diced celery	Oil for frying
1 cup bean sprouts	Chopped green onion or
3 large eggs	sliced almonds, for garnish (optional)

Prepare meat by dicing the chicken or pork or breaking the shrimp and crab into small pieces. Put in a large mixing bowl with the onion, celery, and bean sprouts.

In another bowl, beat the eggs with the salt and soy sauce. Mix into the meat and vegetables.

Heat 1 to 2 tablespoons of oil in a frying pan (if electric, heat to 375°). Ladle in about half the mixture to form 4 small patties. Fry about 2 to 3 minutes on each side. Remove and repeat with the second half, using more oil if necessary.

Serve hot topped with green onion or almonds, if desired. *Makes 4 servings.*

SANDWICHES

CRAB-CHEESE MELT

Serve this open-faced sandwich for an easy and delicious luncheon or supper dish with coleslaw or fresh fruit slices.

12 ounces crabmeat or GF imitation crab
³/4 cup country-style cottage cheese, blended smooth
¹/3 cup mayonnaise
¹/2 cup grated Cheddar cheese
3 green onions, sliced thin

5 drops Tabasco sauce
2 teaspoons Worcestershire sauce or 1 teaspoon GF soy sauce
6 Crumpets (page 75) or Australian Toaster Buns (page 76) or 12 slices GF bread

Preheat oven to 400°.

Break the crab into bite-sized pieces. Set aside.

In a medium mixing bowl, mix together the cottage cheese and mayonnaise. Stir in the Cheddar cheese, onions, Tabasco sauce, and Worcestershire sauce. Gently fold in the crab pieces.

Split the 6 muffins and divide the crab mixture on the 12 pieces. Place on a large baking sheet and bake for 10 to 12 minutes. *Makes 12 open-faced sandwiches.*

GYROS SANDWICH

A great party sandwich and different. *In Greece the pita bread might be stuffed with mounds of thinly sliced, slowly grilled lamb, yogurt, and cucumbers. This more modest version uses seasoned ground lamb broiled or grilled slowly on a barbecue. You may moisten your pita bread with yogurt or, for the lactose intolerant, substitute some of the Double Dill Dip (page 199) made with nondairy sour cream. You will need four pitas.*

1 pound ground lamb
1/2 pound mild pork
  sausage
3 cloves garlic, crushed
1 tablespoon lemon juice
1/2 teaspoon salt
1/2 teaspoon pepper
1 teaspoon oregano,
  crushed fine

1 teaspoon crushed basil
Garnish (optional): yogurt
  or Double Dill Dip,
  thinned; sliced onions;
  grated cucumber or
  alfalfa sprouts; sliced
  tomatoes

Mix together the lamb, pork, garlic, lemon juice, salt, pepper, oregano, and basil. Mold into thin patties. Broil the patties in the oven 7 inches from the heat or grill on a not-too-hot barbecue until the meat is cooked through. The ingredients can be prepared ahead of time and the cooking done after the guests arrive.

Slit the pitas and fill with the desired condiments plus the meat patty or patties (if you make them small, as I do). *Makes 4 servings.*

BETTE'S SPECIAL FILLED BUNS

These buns cooked with their own meat filling are flavored with a hint of the Far East. These bear little resemblance to the heavy pastie that, for generations, was carried into the tin mines in old Cornwall as a midday meal. Eat these fresh from the oven or make ahead, refrigerate or freeze, and reheat in the microwave for a special luncheon. They are delicious either way. After you cook the filling recipe, mix up the crumpet dough.

Filling

1 pound lean, boneless pork or boned and skinned chicken breast
1 clove garlic, minced
1/4 teaspoon fresh grated gingerroot
2 teaspoons sugar
2 tablespoons soy sauce, divided

1 1/2 teaspoons cornstarch
1 1/2 teaspoons sherry
1/8 cup water
1 1/2 teaspoons oil, for frying
1/2 medium onion, chopped

1 double recipe Crumpet dough (page 75)

Filling: Cut the meat into small pieces (1/2 inch or less). Place in a small bowl with the garlic, gingerroot, sugar, and 1 tablespoon of the soy sauce.

In another bowl, combine the cornstarch, remaining 1 tablespoon soy sauce, sherry, and the water.

In a wok or frying pan, heat the oil. Add the meat and stir-fry until browned, about 5 minutes. Add the onion and cook together until onion is soft and clear. Stir in the cornstarch mixture and cook, stirring, until sauce boils and thickens. Set aside to cool.

Buns: Make a double recipe of Crumpet dough. Prepare muffin rings as for crumpets but, using only half the dough, divide among the 12 rings. Spread the dough with a spatula evenly over the bottom. Divide the filling and put about 2 tablespoons on the center of each bun. Spread, but don't let the filling touch the edges of the rings. Top with remaining dough and spread gently over the filling. Cover and let rise until doubled in bulk, 40 to 45 minutes for regular yeast; 20 to 25 minutes for rapid-rise yeast.

Bake in a preheated 375° oven for 20 to 25 minutes. Serve hot. *Makes 12 buns.*

CASSEROLES

JEANNE'S INCREDIBLE TURKEY CASSEROLE

So easy, so good, and made in minutes, this turkey or chicken pie has a crust poured on as batter. No rolling and cutting. Use a deep casserole for a thick crust; a flat one for a thinner crust. This recipe was adapted with permission of the Portland/Vancouver Chapter of GIG.

2 cups cooked poultry	3/4 teaspoon poultry
1 cup diced carrots	seasoning
1/2 cup frozen peas	3/4 teaspoon salt, or to
1/2 cup thin-sliced celery	taste
1/4 cup chopped onion	Dash pepper
1/2 cup chicken broth or	4 eggs
water	1 tablespoon margarine,
1 cup GF flour mix	melted
1/2 teaspoon baking	1 cup milk or nondairy
powder	liquid

Preheat oven to 375°.

Cube the turkey or chicken. Set aside.

In a medium saucepan, place the carrots, peas, celery, onion, and chicken broth. Bring to a boil, lower to a simmer. Cook 5 minutes. Add the poultry and cook until heated through. Pour into a buttered 2-quart casserole.

In a medium mixing bowl, blend the flour, baking powder, poultry seasoning, salt, and pepper. Add the eggs, margarine, and milk.

Beat with hand mixer for about 1 minute. Pour over the meat and vegetables. Bake for 30 to 35 minutes until the crust is firm and browned. *Makes 4 or 5 servings.*

AUSTRIAN CHEESE PUFF

An elegant but filling soufflé for luncheon or supper. You can use leftover vegetables or freshly cooked ones for this soufflé. Try to use one green vegetable with one white or colored one. If desired, prepare the soufflé ahead, refrigerate, and bake just before guests arrive.

$1/4$ cup plus 2 tablespoons butter	$1/8$ teaspoon nutmeg
1 cup fresh mushrooms, sliced	$1/4$ cup rice flour
	$1/2$ cup grated Swiss cheese
5 eggs, separated	$1^1/4$ cups cauliflower or broccoli florets, cooked
$1/2$ cup sour cream or nondairy substitute	1 cup peas, asparagus, or carrots, cooked
$1/2$ teaspoon salt, or to taste	$3/4$ cup cooked ham, poultry, or sausage
Dash pepper	

Preheat oven to 350°.

In 1 tablespoon of the butter sauté the mushrooms until golden. Set aside.

In a medium mixing bowl, beat $1/4$ cup of the butter with the egg yolks, one at a time. Add the sour cream, salt, pepper, and nutmeg. Gradually add the flour and half the cheese.

In a large mixing bowl, beat the egg whites until stiff. Fold in the egg yolk mixture. Pour half the mixture into a buttered 10″ × 6″ casserole. Top with half the vegetables and half the meat. Sprinkle on half of the remaining cheese. Pour on the rest of the soufflé mixture.

Top with the remaining vegetables and meat. Sprinkle on the last of the cheese. Dot with the remaining tablespoon of butter. Bake for 35 minutes until firm and brown on top. *Makes 6 servings.*

SAUSAGE AND CHEESE STRATA

An easy luncheon or supper dish that can be prepared the night before or up to 3 hours before serving. Team with a tossed salad or a spicy slaw for a full meal. For dessert, add fresh or canned fruit. For a very different strata, see Vegetable and Cheese Strata (page 244).

1/2 pound pork sausage
8 green onions, sliced
  (1/4 cup)
2 cups grated Cheddar
  cheese

1/2 teaspoon prepared
  mustard
3 cups GF bread cubes
11/2 cups milk
4 eggs, beaten

In a large frying pan, brown the sausage. Drain. Add the green onions and cook until clear. Set aside to cool; stir in the cheese, mustard, and bread cubes. Place in an 8″ square buttered casserole.

Beat together the milk and eggs, and pour them over the casserole. Cover and refrigerate from 3 hours to overnight.

Preheat oven to 350°. Bake, uncovered, for 50 to 55 minutes, or until golden brown. Let stand a few minutes before serving. *Makes 6 servings.*

CREAMED DISH

CHICKEN À LA KING

An old favorite using leftovers to create a new dish, now updated and gluten free. Serve this in the Potato Baskets (page 240), on Crumpets (page 75), or GF toast points. The mushrooms are optional.

3 tablespoons butter or margarine
1 1/2 tablespoons minced green onion
2 tablespoons sweet rice flour
1 1/2 cups chicken broth
2 cups cooked chicken, diced

One 4-ounce can mushrooms, drained (optional)
2 tablespoons diced pimiento
1 to 2 tablespoons golden sherry

In a 2-quart saucepan, melt the butter, add onions, then stir in the flour and cook over low heat until mixed. Add the broth; simmer, stirring occasionally, until thickened.

When the sauce is cooked, add the chicken, mushrooms if desired, pimiento, and sherry. Simmer until well blended before filling the potato baskets or spooning over crumpets or toast points. *Makes 6 servings.*

LUNCHEON SALAD

TACO SALAD

A full-meal salad to be made on individual plates, this is one of my summer favorites. The ingredients listed below will make a large serving. Increase the amounts as desired for the number of salads you wish to make. For a fresher taste, replace taco seasoning with fresh GF taco salsa. Serve with GF taco chips.

1/3 pound lean ground beef	3 tablespoons grated Cheddar cheese
2 teaspoons water	1 tablespoon ripe olives (optional)
2 teaspoons GF taco seasoning mix	1 small tomato, cut in wedges or diced
1 cup shredded iceberg lettuce	1/2 small avocado
1 tablespoon chopped onion	1 tablespoon mayonnaise
	Dash Tabasco sauce

Brown the ground beef in a small skillet. When cooked, add the water and taco seasoning mix. Let simmer while preparing the other ingredients.

Spread the lettuce on a large plate. Sprinkle on the onion. Top with the meat, then cheese, and olives (if used). Place the tomato wedges around the outside or, if diced, sprinkle them over the salad.

Peel and pit the avocado; place in small bowl and mash. Mix in the mayonnaise and add the Tabasco sauce. Use this dressing as a dollop on top of the salad. *Enough for 1 large serving.*

MEATS

CASSEROLES

Moussaka
Russian Cabbage Rolls
Shepherd's Pie
Bobotie (Beef Casserole)
Meatballs Mole

STOVE-TOP DISHES

Java Beef with Pineapple
   Sauce
Hungarian Goulash
Easy Swiss Steak
Beef Curry with Vegetables
Ginger Beef
   Ginger Beef with Chinese
     Pea Pods
Pork with Vegetables

Pork Cutlets with Apple-
   Brandy Sauce

SAUCES FOR MEAT

Spiced Cranberry Sauce
Orange-Raisin Sauce

SEE ALSO

Quiche with a Hash Brown
   Crust
Gyros Sandwich
Bette's Special Filled Buns
Austrian Cheese Puff
Sausage and Cheese Strata
Taco Salad

The celiac diet does not forbid meats *unless* they are breaded, stuffed, gravied, marinated, or (horrors!) basted with gluten-laced bouillon. And most of us have learned, to our dismay, that we can never safely order a meat casserole when dining out. Even though most of the ingredients sound safe, the liquid may be bouillon and the thickening will almost always be wheat flour.

But we can serve meat dishes in our own homes. Meat as the main dish in a meal is not as popular in other cultures as in the United States; but many nationalities have created wonderful dishes using less meat or the inexpensive cuts. This section includes a wide variety of recipes using meat in casseroles, pies, curries, and stir-frys, which I've adapted to fit our dietary limitations.

Try them, varying the seasonings to your family's taste, and, next time you dine out and order the plainest meat on the menu, don't let your companions feel sorry for you. Tell them of that tasty casserole you're planning to create for the next meal at home and of the dozen others you enjoy.

CASSEROLES

MOUSSAKA

I first tasted this version of moussaka in a remote Greek inn in early spring when eggplant was out of season. This casserole takes about 30 minutes to put together, but it can be done ahead of time and baked just before dinner. A delicious change for a company meal calling for only a salad and dessert. You can replace the potato topping with the more traditional large eggplant cut into ¹/₂-inch-thick slices. If desired, this may be served with the Tomato Sauce from page 254, but I usually serve the moussaka plain.

Filling

2 tablespoons olive oil
1¹/₂ pounds ground beef or
   lamb or a combination
   of the two
1 medium onion, chopped
One 14-ounce jar GF
   spaghetti sauce
¹/₂ cup red wine or beef
   broth
1 teaspoon dried parsley
   flakes
1 teaspoon salt
¹/₂ teaspoon pepper
¹/₄ teaspoon nutmeg
1 cup grated Parmesan
   cheese
²/₃ cup dry GF bread
   crumbs
1 egg, beaten

Topping

1¹/₂ cups water
¹/₃ cup milk
2¹/₂ tablespoons butter or
   margarine
¹/₂ teaspoon salt
1¹/₂ cups Potato Buds

White Sauce

¹/₄ cup margarine or butter
¹/₄ cup rice flour
³/₄ teaspoon salt
¹/₄ teaspoon nutmeg
2 cups milk or nondairy
   liquid
2 eggs, slightly beaten

Preheat oven to 375°.

In a large skillet, heat the oil. Add the meat and chopped onion and cook until meat is lightly browned. Stir in the spaghetti sauce, wine, parsley flakes, salt, pepper, and nutmeg. Bring to a boil, reduce heat to a simmer, and cook, uncovered, until half the liquid is absorbed, about 20 minutes. Meanwhile, prepare the topping and white sauce.

Topping: Heat the water, milk, butter, and salt to boiling. Remove from heat and stir in the Potato Buds until liquid is absorbed. Form into a loaf on wax paper; cool until ready to use. Cut into slices 1/2-inch thick.

Sauce: In a 2-quart saucepan, melt the margarine over low heat. Blend together the flour, salt, and nutmeg; add to the margarine until smooth and bubbly. Stir in the milk and heat to boiling, stirring constantly. Boil for 1 minute to thicken. Combine about 1/2 cup of the hot mixture with the eggs. Blend back into the hot sauce and remove from heat.

Stir 2/3 cup of the Parmesan cheese and 1/3 cup of the bread crumbs plus the egg into the meat mixture. Remove from heat.

Sprinkle the remaining bread crumbs in a greased 9" × 13 1/2" baking dish. Spread the meat mixture over the bread crumbs and sprinkle with 2 tablespoons of the remaining cheese. Top with a layer of the mashed potato slices and then pour the white sauce over the casserole. Top with the remaining cheese.

Cook, uncovered, for 45 minutes. Let stand for about 15 minutes before cutting into squares for serving. *Serves 6 to 8.*

RUSSIAN CABBAGE ROLLS

In spite of its peasant beginnings, this can be a company dish. Easily made ahead and refrigerated, it allows the hostess time with the guests while the casserole is cooking. Serve it with a green salad and either buttered noodles or little red potatoes boiled in their jackets.

1 head green cabbage

Filling

1/2 pound lean ground beef
1/2 pound ground pork or
   mild pork sausage
1 tablespoon minced onion
1 cup cooked brown or
   white rice
1 teaspoon salt
1/4 teaspoon lemon pepper
Dash garlic salt

1/4 teaspoon dry mustard
One 8-ounce can tomato
   sauce

Sauce

1 1/2 tablespoons rice flour
1/2 teaspoon salt
1 1/2 cups plain yogurt

Chopped chives, for
   garnish

Preheat oven to 375°.

Blanch cabbage in boiling water for 5 minutes. Remove from kettle and let drain and cool. Remove the large outer leaves carefully after removing the core.

In a large bowl, mix together the meats, onion, rice, salt, lemon pepper, garlic salt, and mustard. Slowly add the tomato sauce until the mixture is moist enough to stick together well, using about two-thirds of the sauce.

Place 1 heaping tablespoon of filling in center of each leaf (the extra large outside ones may be divided into two), tuck leaf edges over the filling, and roll. Place the packages, seam side down, in a 10″ × 10″ or 9″ × 12″ baking dish. You should have about 12.

Mix the rice flour and salt with yogurt. Pour the sauce over the rolls. Cover and bake for 1 1/2 hours, removing cover for the last 1/2 hour of baking. Garnish with chopped chives before serving. *Makes 4 to 5 servings.*

SHEPHERD'S PIE

This stew with a potato topping was one of my mother's "reserve" recipes when faced with unexpected company on the farm. With the nearest store miles away, she had to use vegetables from the garden plus hamburger from the freezer. I've simplified some of her fresh ingredients to items you'll have on your shelf. This hearty meal in a dish can be prepared ahead and baked later or put together easily at dinnertime.

2 pounds lean ground beef
1 tablespoon rice flour
1 tablespoon vegetable oil
1 medium white onion,
 diced
4 green onions, sliced thin
1 cup diced carrots
3/4 cup diced celery
1 teaspoon parsley flakes
1 teaspoon salt, or to taste
Pepper to taste
1 tablespoon
 Worcestershire sauce
3/4 cup tomato sauce

3/4 cup beef stock
3/4 cup frozen peas

Topping

2 cups water
1/2 cup milk
3 tablespoons butter or
 margarine
3/4 teaspoon salt
2 cups Potato Buds

1/2 cup grated Cheddar
 cheese (optional)

Preheat oven to 350°.

Coat a heavy skillet with nonstick vegetable spray and brown the beef over medium heat. Stir in rice flour and remove to a dish.

In the same skillet, heat the oil and add the white onion, green onion, carrot, and celery. Turn heat to low and simmer, covered, for about 20 minutes, or until the vegetables are tender. If there is not enough liquid, add a tablespoon of water.

To the cooked vegetables add the meat, parsley, salt, pepper, Worcestershire sauce, tomato sauce, and beef stock. Stir and pour into a 2-quart casserole. Cover and bake for 20 minutes while you make the topping.

Topping: Prepare Potato Buds as directed on package, using the quantities listed above. Set aside.

Stir the frozen peas into the meat mixture and spread the mashed potatoes on top. Turn up oven to 375° and bake for 45 minutes more, topping with the cheese (if desired) during the last 5 minutes. *Makes 4 or 5 servings.*

BOBOTIE (Beef Casserole)

This fruited beef dish with a custard topping is a special treat from South Africa. The wonderful blending of meat, fruit, and spice is a heritage of the early Dutch settlers. I've given a large recipe here, but you can halve all but the topping ingredients. Serve with rice or, as the Afrikaners do, with corn grits.

2 medium onions, chopped	2 tablespoons sugar
2 tablespoons margarine or butter	2 tablespoons lemon juice
2 pounds extra-lean ground beef	1 tablespoon curry powder
1 egg	2 teaspoons salt
3/4 cup milk	1/4 teaspoon pepper
2 slices GF bread, cubed	
1/4 cup dried apricots, chopped fine	*Topping*
1/4 cup raisins	1 egg
2 tablespoons blanched almonds, chopped fine	3/4 cup milk or nondairy liquid
	1/4 teaspoon turmeric

Preheat oven to 350°.

In a large skillet, sauté the onion in the margarine until transparent. Add the ground beef and cook until browned. Remove from heat.

In a large mixing bowl, combine the egg, milk, and bread cubes. Let set for a few minutes and then mash the bread with a fork. Add the apricots, raisins, almonds, sugar, lemon juice, curry, salt, and pepper. Mix until well blended. Add the meat mixture and blend. Pour into a 2 1/2-quart casserole, pressing lightly. Bake for 30 minutes before adding the topping.

While this is baking, in a small bowl, beat the egg with the milk and turmeric until just blended. When the casserole has cooked for 30 minutes, remove from the oven and pour this custard over it. Return to the oven and bake for 10 to 15 minutes, or until topping is set. *Makes 8 servings.*

MEATBALLS MOLE

Don't pass up this excitingly different flavor in meatballs. The chocolate in the sauce spells Mexico. The Pre-Columbian Indians used chocolate as a spice long before the Europeans started adding sugar and making chocolate desserts. Serve with rice or spaghetti.

Meatballs

1 pound lean ground beef
1 egg, beaten
1/2 cup milk or nondairy
  liquid
3/4 cup crushed corn chips
1 teaspoon salt
2 1/2 teaspoons rice flour
2 tablespoons vegetable oil

Sauce

3 medium onions, chopped
1 clove garlic, minced

2 tablespoons sugar
1 tablespoon chili powder
1 teaspoon ground cumin
1 teaspoon ground
  coriander
1 teaspoon dried oregano
1 1/2 teaspoons salt
One 16-ounce can tomato
  puree
1 square unsweetened
  chocolate
1 cup water

Meatballs: In a large mixing bowl, combine the beef, egg, milk, corn chips, and salt. Mix until well combined. Refrigerate 1 hour.
Preheat oven to 350°.
Shape the mixture into 20 balls. Place flour in low, flat pan and roll the balls in it until coated (reserve remaining flour).
In a large skillet or heavy Dutch oven, heat the oil and brown the meatballs, a few at a time. Remove as they brown to a 2 1/2-quart casserole.

Sauce: In the same pan, sauté the onion and garlic until translucent. Remove pan from heat.

Combine the sugar, chili powder, cumin, coriander, oregano, salt, and the flour that remained from rolling the meatballs. Stir into the skillet along with the tomato puree, chocolate, and the water.

Return to heat and bring mixture to boiling, stirring constantly. Reduce heat to a simmer, cover, and cook for 30 minutes, stirring occasionally. Pour the sauce over the meatballs in the casserole and bake, covered, for 45 minutes (see Note). *Makes 4 to 6 servings.*

NOTE: If you prefer, you may add the meatballs to the sauce in the skillet or Dutch oven and simmer, covered, for 30 minutes.

STOVE-TOP DISHES

JAVA BEEF WITH PINEAPPLE SAUCE

Sweet, sour, and spicy. A wonderful touch to that inexpensive pot roast. Serve with white rice and tropical fruit to complement the sweet-spicy flavor of the meat.

2¹/₂ pounds boneless beef pot roast
1 tablespoon vegetable oil
2 cloves garlic, minced
¹/₂ cup chopped onion
One 8-ounce can pineapple juice
1¹/₂ cups water
¹/₂ cup GF soy sauce

¹/₄ cup dry sherry
2¹/₂ tablespoons brown sugar
1 tablespoon fresh gingerroot, grated
1 teaspoon allspice
2 cinnamon sticks, broken
4 teaspoons cornstarch

Trim excess fat from beef, wash, and pat dry.

In a large pot or Dutch oven, heat the oil. Add the garlic and onion and sauté for about 1 minute. Add the beef and brown on each side.

Combine the pineapple juice, water, soy sauce, sherry, sugar, gingerroot, allspice, and cinnamon. Pour over the roast. Bring to a boil; reduce heat and simmer for 1 1/2 to 2 hours, turning occasionally.

Remove the meat from the pot. Strain 1 cup of broth into a small saucepan. Mix the cornstarch with cold water to make a paste. Add a bit of the hot broth and then pour the mixture into the saucepan. Cook, stirring frequently, until clear and thickened.

To serve, slice meat and serve with the gravy. *Makes 6 servings.*

HUNGARIAN GOULASH

A great way to use those tough cuts of meat or to stretch a small amount for a crowd, this dish can be cooked ahead and the yogurt and sour cream added just before serving. The recipe below suggests stove-top cooking, but I often brown the beef and onions in a frying pan and then place the rest of the ingredients, except the sour cream and yogurt, in a slow-cooking electric pot, and leave it to cook all day. Serve with fresh egg noodles (page 228) or with rice.

2 pounds stew meat or sirloin steak	1 1/2 teaspoons salt
1 tablespoon vegetable oil	1/2 teaspoon pepper
1 cup diced onions	1/4 teaspoon ground cloves
1 cup diced carrots	1 tablespoon brown sugar
One 16-ounce can tomatoes	2 tablespoons rice flour
1 cup beef stock	1/4 cup water
1 tablespoon paprika	1/4 cup sour cream or nondairy substitute
	1/4 cup plain yogurt

Cut the stew meat into 1/2-inch slices (or slice the steak into 1/4-inch slices). In a large skillet, brown the beef quickly. Remove the meat from the skillet, then add the oil and sauté the onion until clear.

Return the beef to the skillet (or place it in your electric pot). Add the carrots, tomatoes, beef stock, paprika, salt, pepper, cloves, and sugar. Combine the rice flour with the water and stir in. Cover and let simmer until the meat is tender, 20 minutes to an hour. Longer cooking seems to increase the flavor (in a Crock-Pot this can be several hours on High or all day on Low).

Just before serving, stir in the sour cream and yogurt and heat through. *Makes 6 to 8 servings.*

EASY SWISS STEAK

I've been making this easy top-of-the-stove version of Swiss steak for years. After I was put on a gluten-free diet, it took only a change in flours to continue this family favorite. One tester suggests adding chopped onion as you brown the last of the meat. Serve with fluffy mashed potatoes.

2½ pounds beef round steak
¼ cup plus 2 tablespoons rice flour
½ teaspoon onion salt
2 tablespoons vegetable oil plus fat trimmed from steak
⅓ cup ketchup

3 cups beef broth or water
2 to 4 tablespoons red wine or 1 tablespoon wine vinegar
Salt and pepper to taste
1 to 2 tablespoons chopped onion (optional)

Wash beef, pat dry, and trim off fat. Cut meat into 2½-by-2½-inch sections. Coat the pieces with ¼ cup of the flour and onion salt; gently pound. If desired, add some salt and pepper to the flour.

Heat the oil plus fat in a Dutch oven or large skillet. Brown meat a few pieces at a time. When all are browned, remove the fat and return meat to the pan. Add the ketchup, broth, and wine to almost cover meat. If needed, add water. Bring to a boil, reduce heat to simmer, and cook for 2½ to 3 hours. Season to taste with salt and pepper.

When done, the meat should be very tender and the stock slightly thickened.

Make a paste of the 2 tablespoons rice flour and broth. Add, a little at a time, to the broth, thickening to your taste. *Makes 6 servings.*

BEEF CURRY WITH VEGETABLES

This mild South African curry is quick cooking and easy to make. It is very popular with my testers for it can make a new dish of leftover cooked beef and carrots. I don't usually serve any condiment with this except chopped green onion tops for a dash of fresh color.

6 tablespoons margarine	4 teaspoons curry powder
1 cup sliced fresh mushrooms	1 teaspoon grated fresh gingerroot
1/2 cup chopped onion	2 cups beef broth
1 clove garlic, minced	2 to 3 cups cooked beef
4 tablespoons rice flour	1 cup cooked carrots
1 teaspoon salt, or to taste	1 cup sour cream or nondairy substitute
2 tablespoons sugar, or to taste	

In a large skillet, melt the margarine. Add the mushrooms, onion, and garlic; sauté until the onions are clear.

Combine the rice flour, salt, sugar, curry powder, and grated gingerroot. Add to the sautéed vegetables. Slowly add the beef broth, stirring constantly. Bring to a boil and simmer until thickened.

Add the meat and carrots and cook on low heat until they are heated through. Add the sour cream and stir until blended and warm. Serve immediately with white rice. *Makes 6 servings.*

GINGER BEEF

A simple, inexpensive dish with a delicate blend of oriental flavors, this easy stir-fry, unlike many oriental dishes, can remain on the stove over very low heat until the hostess is ready to serve. Pair with white rice and fruit for a tasty meal.

1 pound sirloin steak	2 teaspoons cornstarch
6 drops sesame oil	2/3 cup beef stock
1 tablespoon vegetable oil	2 tablespoons GF soy
1 1/2 cloves garlic, minced	sauce
2 tablespoons fresh	1 teaspoon rice wine or
gingerroot, grated	1 tablespoon white wine
2 teaspoons sugar	4 green onions, sliced thin

Slice steak into razor-thin strips. Prepare or measure all other ingredients. Heat skillet and add sesame and vegetable oils. Fry meat on high or medium-high heat for a couple of minutes, until the pink is gone and the steak juices have diluted the oil. Remove the meat to a bowl with a slotted spoon.

Into the steak juice drop the garlic and gingerroot. Stir. Combine the sugar and cornstarch and add to the juice. Stir again and pour in the beef stock. Add the soy sauce and wine and cook until sauce thickens. Return the cooked steak to the pan.

Cook for about 3 minutes. Dish up immediately or leave on simmer until ready to serve. Put in a bowl and garnish with the sliced green onions. *Makes 4 or 5 servings.*

GINGER BEEF WITH CHINESE PEA PODS: Omit the green onion garnish, and add, after the meat is returned to the skillet, one 10-ounce package frozen Chinese pea pods or 1/2 pound of fresh Chinese pea pods and 1/2 cup slivered blanched almonds.

Cook until the pea pods are just tender. Serve immediately. The pea pods cannot stand without wilting. *Makes 6 servings.*

PORK WITH VEGETABLES

An easy top-of-the-stove combination to serve as a stew on mashed potatoes or noodles. You can make this ahead; it's even better the next day.

1 pound lean boneless
   pork
2 tablespoons vegetable oil
1 clove garlic, minced
1 tablespoon minced fresh
   parsley
1³/₄ cups chicken broth
¹/₄ cup dry white wine
¹/₄ teaspoon dried thyme
¹/₄ teaspoon powdered bay
   leaf
¹/₈ teaspoon pepper
8 to 10 small boiling
   onions, peeled

2 cups carrots, in ¹/₂-inch
   chunks
1 cup fresh button
   mushrooms or one
   4-ounce can drained
   mushrooms
¹/₄ cup rice flour
¹/₂ cup cold water
¹/₄ cup cream or nondairy
   liquid, undiluted
1¹/₂ tablespoons lemon
   juice

Cut the pork into 1-inch cubes. Brown them in hot oil in a Dutch oven. Stir in the garlic and parsley, then add the chicken broth and white wine. Bring to a boil. Add the thyme, bay leaf, and pepper. Reduce heat to a simmer, cover the pork mixture, and cook for about 45 minutes.

Add the onions, carrots, and mushrooms. Bring to a boil again and then reduce to a simmer. Cook until carrots are tender crisp, about 15 minutes.

Combine the flour and water. Sir into the stew and cook until thickened. Add the cream and lemon juice. *Makes 4 servings.*

PORK CUTLETS WITH
APPLE-BRANDY SAUCE

In this wonderful quick-to-fix pork dish, ingredients can be altered to fit the seasons or your palate. You can use frozen orange juice concentrate instead of brandy, a garlic clove instead of the minced onions, pear or Chinese pear instead of apple. Serve with either white rice or small red potatoes.

1 pound lean pork cutlets	1 teaspoon dried thyme
Salt and pepper to taste	3 tablespoons red wine
1 1/2 tablespoons vegetable	vinegar
oil	3/4 cup chicken broth
1 1/2 tablespoons margarine	1 tablespoon brandy or
or butter	frozen orange juice
	concentrate
Sauce	1 tablespoon brown sugar
1 cup thinly sliced apples	Orange slices for garnish
2 tablespoons minced	(optional)
onion	

Place the cutlets between two sheets of aluminum foil or wax paper and flatten using a rolling pin. Season with the salt and pepper. In a large skillet, heat the oil and margarine. Add the cutlets and cook over medium heat until brown and just cooked through, about 2 minutes per side. Remove to a serving dish.

Add the apple slices and onion to the drippings in pan. Sauté until the onion is clear, about 3 minutes. Add the thyme and vinegar and cook for about 30 seconds. Add the chicken broth, brandy, and sugar. Simmer for a few minutes.

Return the cutlets to the sauce and simmer until they are heated through. Arrange meat on the serving dish and pour sauce over it. Garnish, if desired, with split and twisted orange slices. *Makes 4 servings.*

SAUCES FOR MEAT

SPICED CRANBERRY SAUCE

A spicy fruit sauce to dress up that plain pork roast, baked ham, or Turkey Loaf (page 308). Made easily in less than 10 minutes with a can of cranberries and spices from your shelf.

One 8-ounce can whole
   cranberry sauce
1 tablespoon butter or
   margarine
1¹/₂ teaspoons brown
   sugar

1¹/₂ teaspoons horseradish
¹/₄ teaspoon dry mustard
¹/₈ teaspoon allspice

Place all ingredients in a small saucepan and heat to boiling, stirring occasionally. Reduce heat and simmer 5 minutes. *Makes 1 cup.*

ORANGE-RAISIN SAUCE

A simple, easy-to-make fruit sauce that enhances the flavor of pork or ham.

$1/2$ cup raisins	Dash of salt
$1/2$ cup water	$1/8$ teaspoon allspice
$1/3$ cup currant jelly	1 tablespoon cornstarch
$1/2$ teaspoon dried orange peel or 1 teaspoon fresh grated orange zest	$1/3$ cup orange juice

In a saucepan, heat the raisins, water, jelly, orange peel, salt, and allspice.

Meanwhile, mix together the cornstarch and orange juice, and add them to the raisin mixture when it reaches boiling. Stir until thickened and clear. *Makes 1 1/2 cups.*

POULTRY

CASSEROLES (Chicken)

Lucile's Chicken (or Rabbit)
　　Ragout
Chicken in Asparagus Sauce
Tandoori-style Chicken
Sherried Chicken with Rice

STOVE-TOP CHICKEN

Chicken in Coconut Sauce
South African Fruited Curry
Moroccan Chicken
Hungarian Chicken

BAKED OR GRILLED
CHICKEN

Haitian Chicken
Teriyaki-style Baked Chicken
Tropical Chicken Breasts
Grandma's Chicken Wings
Hawaiian Chicken Chunks

STIR-FRY CHICKEN

Easy Almond Chicken
Cashew Chicken

TURKEY

Stuffed Turkey Rolls
Turkey Loaf
Mediterranean Meatballs

DRESSING AND SALSA

Cranberry Dressing
Cranberry Salsa

SEE ALSO

Jeanne's Incredible Turkey
　　Casserole
Chicken à la King
Shanghai Chicken Wings

During the Great Depression, we were promised "a chicken in every pot." I can't offer that, but in this chapter I've tried to give you a chicken recipe for every mood.

Some form of fowl is found in almost every country; these recipes mirror the varied tastes of people around the world, from Hungarian Chicken to Mediterranean Meatballs, from a teriyaki of the Orient to a curry from South Africa.

My testers, who were often offered dozens of ways to cook chicken, were most important in the final selection of recipes for this chapter. We kept only the ones they considered "tops."

CASSEROLES (Chicken)

LUCILE'S CHICKEN
(or Rabbit) RAGOUT

An exceptional entrée handed down from a friend's French mother, this ragout makes a full meal when served with some crusty Rapid-Rise French Bread (see page 41) and a tossed salad. This can be made ahead and refrigerated before baking. Allow ten more minutes in the oven if refrigerated.

8 or more pieces chicken or rabbit

2³/₄ cups chicken broth

2 cups carrot chunks

6 to 8 tiny boiling onions, peeled

1 teaspoon salt, or to taste

¹/₂ teaspoon freshly ground pepper

¹/₂ teaspoon poultry seasoning

2¹/₂ tablespoons white rice flour

¹/₄ cup dry white wine

¹/₂ cup cream or nondairy substitute

1 teaspoon dried parsley flakes

One 10-ounce package frozen lima beans, defrosted

Wash the chicken and place it in a greased 9″ × 13″ baking dish. Brown under a broiler, about 5 to 6 minutes each side.

While the chicken is browning, bring the chicken broth to a boil. Add the carrots, onions, salt, pepper, and poultry seasoning. Simmer for 10 minutes.

Blend the rice flour with a few tablespoons of cold water. Stir into the simmering broth and cook until slightly thickened. Remove from heat. Add the wine, cream, and parsley flakes.

Add the lima beans to the chicken, pour the sauce with vegetables over all, and cover with foil. (If making ahead, refrigerate at this point.) Bake in a preheated 350° oven for 1 hour. Remove foil and continue cooking for 15 minutes longer. *Makes 4 or 5 servings.*

CHICKEN IN ASPARAGUS SAUCE

A delicious and different company dinner, and easy enough for a family meal. This casserole can be made ahead and pulled out to bake as the guests (or family) are gathering. Use the whole chicken or, for a more elegant dish, use boneless chicken breasts. Serve with brown rice or small red potatoes. The sauce will be pale green if you use green asparagus, rich cream color if you use white or blanched asparagus.

8 or more pieces uncooked
chicken
2 tablespoons vegetable
oil
1 cup whole skinned
almonds

Sauce

One 12-ounce can
asparagus pieces

2^1/$_4$ tablespoons sweet rice
flour
^{1}/$_2$ teaspoon salt
^{1}/$_4$ teaspoon white pepper
^{1}/$_2$ teaspoon onion powder
^{1}/$_4$ teaspoon garlic powder
2 cups chicken broth
One 6-ounce can
evaporated milk or
^{3}/$_4$ cup nondairy liquid

Preheat oven to 350°.

Wash chicken and pat dry.

In a large skillet heat the oil and brown the chicken on both sides. Remove and arrange in a large, flat baking dish. Pour the almonds into the hot skillet and stir until they start to brown. Sprinkle over the chicken.

Sauce: Drain the asparagus, reserving the liquid. Place the pieces in a blender and puree. Pour the puree plus the reserved liquid into a large saucepan. Add the flour, salt, pepper, and onion and garlic powders. Slowly stir in the chicken broth. Cook over medium high heat, stirring, until it starts to thicken. Add the milk and continue cooking until the sauce thickens slightly. Pour over the chicken in the casserole and bake for about 1 hour (see Note). *Makes 5 or 6 servings.*

NOTE: If making ahead, let sauce cool before pouring over the chicken. Refrigerate until ready to bake.

TANDOORI-STYLE CHICKEN

This modified version of the Indian dish is spicy and flavorful, but the ingredients can be found in any supermarket. A friend raised in India declared this an excellent version, which with brown rice and a salad is good enough for a company dinner. The chicken must marinate at least six hours or overnight before baking, grilling, or broiling.

3 to 3¹/₂ pounds chicken
  thighs, breasts, and legs
1 teaspoon cumin
¹/₂ teaspoon coriander
1 teaspoon paprika
¹/₂ teaspoon ground red
  pepper
1 cup plain yogurt
3 tablespoons lemon juice

1 tablespoon grated fresh
  gingerroot
1 teaspoon minced garlic
1 teaspoon salt
¹/₄ teaspoon red food
  coloring (optional)
Lemon slices, for garnish
  (optional)

Wash chicken, remove skin, and score flesh diagonally ¹/₂ inch deep. Set aside.

In a small frying pan, heat the cumin, coriander, paprika, and pepper over low heat until fragrant, about 1 to 2 minutes. Transfer to a large refrigerator dish. Stir in the yogurt, lemon juice, ginger, garlic, salt, and food coloring (if used). Add the chicken and tumble well. Cover and refrigerate overnight or at least 6 hours.

Remove the chicken from the refrigerator 1 hour before cooking. Bake the chicken in the sauce for about 30 minutes at 350° for a moist chicken. Or grill over a barbecue, turning every 10 minutes until done. Or broil in the oven 5 inches from the heat for 30 minutes, again turning every 10 minutes. Baste each side once with the sauce while grilling or broiling.

Garnish with lemon slices, if desired, and serve with brown rice. *Makes 5 or 6 servings.*

SHERRIED CHICKEN WITH RICE

A baked chicken and rice dish that needs only a salad to complete the meal. It takes a while to assemble, but, once it's in the oven, the cook is free to relax. I prefer to cook chicken with the skin on, but the pieces can be skinned if you prefer.

8 pieces chicken legs or thighs or 2 large chicken breasts, split
1/4 cup rice flour
4 tablespoons butter, divided
1 cup sliced mushrooms
1 cup chopped onion
1/2 cup finely diced celery
3/4 cup cream or nondairy liquid

1/2 teaspoon dry mustard
3/4 teaspoon salt
1/4 teaspoon pepper
2 tablespoons sherry
1 cup white rice, washed
2 cups chicken stock, heated
1/2 cup sliced almonds, for topping

Preheat the oven to 350°.

Wash the chicken and dust it with the flour.

In a large frying pan, heat 2 tablespoons of the butter and brown the chicken on all sides, about 5 minutes. Remove from pan.

Add the remaining 2 tablespoons of the butter to the pan (unless there is enough fat) and sauté the mushrooms for 1 minute. Add the onion and celery. Sauté until onion is clear, about 2 minutes. Blend in the cream, mustard, salt, and pepper. Cook, stirring constantly, until the mixture boils and begins to thicken. Remove from heat and stir in the sherry.

Pour the rice into an 8″ × 12″ buttered baking dish. Cover with the hot chicken stock. Add the chicken and top with the sauce and almonds. Cover with a lid (or aluminum foil) and bake 45 minutes. *Makes 4 servings.*

STOVE-TOP CHICKEN

CHICKEN IN COCONUT SAUCE

Chicken thighs cooked in a fruit and coconut milk sauce similar to curry have a delightfully different taste. Serve them with brown rice and fruit slices for a full meal. If you can't find coconut milk, substitute flaked coconut (about 2 tablespoons) and evaporated milk or nondairy milk substitute (not thinned).

2 pounds chicken thighs, boned and skinned	1 teaspoon grated lime peel
1 tablespoon rice flour	1/2 cup golden raisins
3/4 teaspoon salt	2 tablespoons lime juice
1/4 teaspoon pepper	1 teaspoon grated orange peel
1 tablespoon vegetable oil	2 teaspoons sugar
1/4 cup chopped onion	For garnish if desired:
1 teaspoon minced garlic	fresh papaya slices, fresh
1/2 cup coconut milk	pineapple slices, lime
1/2 cup chicken broth	wedges

Wash chicken and dredge it in flour seasoned with 1/4 teaspoon of the salt and the pepper.

In a large skillet, heat the oil and brown the chicken for 3 to 4 minutes. Add the onion and garlic and cook until translucent.

Combine the coconut milk, chicken broth, lime peel, raisins, lime juice, orange peel, and sugar. Pour over the chicken and cook on low heat, covered, for about 10 minutes, or until the chicken is tender. Leave on heat until ready to serve. Place the chicken on a platter or serving dish and cover with the sauce. Garnish with fruit and lime wedges if desired. *Makes 4 servings.*

SOUTH AFRICAN
FRUITED CURRY

A mild chicken curry sure to please family and friends. If you're "turned off" by a strong curry flavor, you should try this. The readily available ingredients and the short cooking time of about 30 minutes make this a quick and easy supper. Serve with white rice.

2 tablespoons margarine or
  butter
4 chicken breasts, boned,
  skinned, and cut into
  thin strips
1 tablespoon rice flour
1 tablespoon vegetable oil
1 medium onion, chopped
3 cloves garlic, minced
2 tablespoons ginger-curry
  powder

1 tablespoon sugar
1 medium cooking apple,
  diced
$^1/_2$ cup golden raisins
$^1/_4$ cup flaked coconut
  (optional)
One 14$^1/_2$-ounce can
  chicken broth
Salt to taste

In a large, heavy skillet, melt the margarine over medium heat. Add the chicken strips and cook for about 4 minutes, stirring frequently. Add the flour and stir, then remove to a dish.

In the same skillet, place the oil, onion, and garlic. Sauté until translucent. Mix together the ginger-curry powder and sugar, and stir in. Add the apple, raisins, and coconut. Pour in the chicken broth. Bring to a boil and reduce heat to low.

Return the chicken to the skillet and let simmer until the fruit is tender and the sauce is thicker. Salt to taste. *Makes 4 servings.*

MOROCCAN CHICKEN

A deliciously spiced dish of chicken and mild vegetables. Serve with a rice couscous, available from specialty sources (see page 345). As it simmers on the stove, you can imagine all the smells and colors of the Casbah. It makes a good family dish as well as an exciting company dinner.

8 chicken thighs, bone in
Salt to taste
Pepper to taste
1 tablespoon olive oil
1 cup chopped onion
2 cups carrots, in 1/2-inch chunks
2 teaspoons paprika
1 tablespoon fresh gingerroot, grated

1/4 teaspoon turmeric
1/4 teaspoon cinnamon
3 tablespoons lemon juice
1 cup chicken broth
1 tablespoon brown sugar
One 15-ounce can garbanzo beans, drained (optional)

Wash chicken and remove skin. Sprinkle lightly with salt and pepper.

In a large frying pan, heat the oil and brown the chicken on medium-high heat. Remove to a platter.

Place the onion in the pan and sauté at medium heat for about 3 minutes, or until clear. Add the carrots and sauté for another 2 minutes. Sprinkle on the paprika, gingerroot, turmeric, and cinnamon. Stir.

Add the lemon juice, chicken broth, and sugar. Return the chicken to the pan. Bring the broth to a boil and reduce the heat. Cover and simmer for 30 minutes, or until the chicken is fork tender and cooked through. Stir in the garbanzo beans, if used, and heat for about 5 more minutes. Serve over Riz Cous or white rice. *Makes 4 servings.*

HUNGARIAN CHICKEN

For this easy, flavorful chicken dish that makes its own delicious sauce, there is only one pan to wash afterward. Serve with buttered egg noodles (page 228) or white rice and a tossed salad. The yogurt used here would be authentic; for the lactose intolerant, use the nondairy sour cream substitute.

8 pieces chicken, bone in
1 tablespoon butter or
  margarine
1 cup chopped onion
1 teaspoon caraway seed
1 teaspoon garlic salt
1/2 teaspoon dill weed

1/2 teaspoon paprika
1/4 teaspoon pepper
1/2 cup white wine
1 cup plain yogurt or
  nondairy sour cream
  substitute

Wash the chicken and pat dry. In a large skillet, heat the butter. Add the chicken and brown on both sides, about 10 minutes. Add the onion and cook until onion is translucent. Drain excess oil.

Sprinkle chicken with the caraway seed, garlic salt, dill weed, paprika, and pepper, and pour the wine over all. Reduce heat, cover, and simmer for about 25 to 30 minutes, or until the chicken is tender.

Stir the yogurt into the pan and heat (but do not boil). Serve immediately. *Makes 4 servings.*

BAKED OR GRILLED CHICKEN

HAITIAN CHICKEN

Haitian Chicken is easy for the family and great for guests. Serve this tasty baked dish with rice couscous and a fresh fruit salad for a complete meal. Your may use chicken breasts, but I suggest the dark meat because the Caribbean chickens are more gamey tasting, and the flavor of the darker meat blends better with the tangy sauce.

8 to 10 chicken legs or thighs
3/4 cup chopped sweet pickles (page 252; see Note)
1/4 cup sweet pickle juice (page 252)
1/3 cup ketchup
1/4 cup GF soy sauce
1/2 cup brown sugar

Preheat oven to 400°.

Wash and place the chicken pieces on vegetable oil–sprayed aluminum foil in a 9″ × 13″ baking dish. Bake for 20 to 25 minutes, or until the skin is brown and bubbly.

While the chicken is baking, make a sauce by combining the pickles, juice, ketchup, soy sauce, and sugar (see Note). Heat until just boiling. Remove from stove.

Remove the chicken from the oven and cover liberally with sauce. Reduce heat to 325°. Return pan to oven and let bake about 10 minutes longer. *Makes 4 or 5 servings.*

NOTE: If desired, increase the amount of sauce and serve over white rice instead of couscous by reheating the remaining sauce to serve with the rice.

TERIYAKI-STYLE
BAKED CHICKEN

I like to use chicken thighs for this dish, but you may use split Cornish hens, chicken breasts, or a combination of leg and thigh pieces. The flavor is improved if you leave the bone in. This must marinate at least six hours. Serve with a brown rice pilaf, Ginger Rice (page 219), or white rice.

3 pounds chicken pieces
1/2 cup Chinese cooking
　　wine or medium white
　　wine
1/2 cup chicken broth

1/2 cup GF soy sauce
1 tablespoon brown sugar
1 tablespoon fresh
　　gingerroot, grated

Wash the chicken pieces and place in a baking dish large enough for them to be arranged in no more than 2 layers.

Mix the wine, chicken broth, soy sauce, sugar, and gingerroot. Pour over the chicken. Cover and marinate in the refrigerator for 6 to 8 hours or overnight, turning if top pieces are not covered.

Bake, uncovered, in the marinade, in a preheated 325° oven for 45 minutes. *Makes 6 to 8 servings.*

TROPICAL CHICKEN BREASTS

A moist, spicy chicken dish put together in a few minutes, this can be prepared ahead and popped into the oven about thirty-five minutes before dinner. Serve with plain white rice to enjoy the full ginger-fruit flavor of the chicken and the accompanying fruits.

6 large chicken breast halves, boned and skinned
3 tablespoons lime juice
2 tablespoons candied ginger, minced
1 fresh pineapple, peeled, cored, and sliced

¹/₄ cup dried coconut
3 bananas, peeled and quartered
2 oranges, peeled and sliced

Preheat oven to 400°.

Wash chicken breasts and pat dry. Arrange them in a single layer in a 9″ × 13″ pan or casserole.

In a blender or food processor, whirl together the lime juice, ginger, and 1 slice of the pineapple. Spoon the mixture over the chicken. Bake for approximately 35 minutes, or until chicken is tender. When chicken is done, sprinkle with the coconut and broil for a minute or so, until the sauce is bubbling and the coconut is lightly browned. Watch for burning.

Meanwhile, place bananas, oranges, and remaining pineapple in another 9″ × 13″ dish; they can overlap. (Put a little of the pineapple juice or a squirt of lemon over the bananas to keep them from turning dark.)

Transfer the chicken to the center of a large serving platter. Pour the pan juices over the fruit and broil for 1 to 2 minutes. Place the fruit around the chicken and serve immediately. *Makes 6 servings.*

GRANDMA'S CHICKEN WINGS

When she served these at a Gluten Intolerance Group picnic, Sue, the president, was mobbed for the recipe. With the permission of her ninety-seven-year-old grandmother, she shares the recipe for this cookbook. These chicken wings are a bit messy to make, but well worthwhile. Disjointed wings without tips can be found in five-pound bags in the frozen foods section of most grocery stores. This recipe can easily be halved.

5 pounds of chicken wings, disjointed, or chicken wing drumettes
Garlic salt to taste
1 cup cornstarch
3 eggs, beaten
2 tablespoons vegetable oil, for frying

$1/2$ cup chicken broth
$1/3$ cup ketchup
$1 1/4$ cups loosely packed brown sugar
2 tablespoons GF soy sauce
$3/4$ cup cider vinegar

Preheat oven to 300°.

Wash the chicken wings and sprinkle with garlic salt. Roll them in the cornstarch, then the beaten eggs. Fry in small batches in hot oil until browned. Remove to a baking dish large enough to hold them all.

In a medium saucepan, mix together the chicken broth, ketchup, brown sugar, soy sauce, and vinegar. Heat to dissolve. Pour over the chicken wings. Bake, lightly covered with aluminum foil, for $1 1/2$ hours, basting or turning often. Serve hot or cold. *Makes 10 to 12 servings.*

HAWAIIAN CHICKEN CHUNKS

Easy-to-prepare chicken breasts or thighs with a sweet, crunchy crust are wonderful with Curried Rice (page 221) or with plain brown rice and a green salad. Prepare ahead and bake later, if desired.

2 whole chicken breasts or 4 thighs, skinned and boned	1 egg, beaten
Salt to taste or lemon juice	1/4 teaspoon powdered ginger
1/4 cup frozen orange juice concentrate, thawed	1/2 cup crushed Kenmai Rice Bran (see Note)
	1/3 cup dried coconut

Preheat oven to 375°.

Wash the chicken breasts and cut each into 4 chunks (cut thighs in half). Salt to taste or sprinkle on lemon juice for flavor.

In a medium bowl, mix the orange juice, egg, and ginger.

In a flat dish, combine the Kenmai Rice Bran and the coconut (for a finer crust, I whirl the coconut in my food processor for a few seconds).

Dip the chicken in the liquid combination and then roll in the crumb mixture. Place in a single layer in an aluminum foil–lined 9″ × 13″ baking pan. Bake, uncovered, for about 35 minutes, or until the chicken is cooked through and the crust is brown. (If browning too much, cover at end of baking.) *Makes 3 or 4 servings.*

NOTE: For a change, replace Kenmai Rice Bran with 1/2 cup popcorn flour (see the list of suppliers on pages 343–347).

APPETIZERS: For a wonderfully easy appetizer, cut the chicken pieces into bite-sized chunks. Bake for 15 to 20 minutes, or until cooked through. Serve hot or cold with a dipping sauce (pages 199–200).

STIR-FRY CHICKEN

EASY ALMOND CHICKEN

This traditional oriental dish can become a cook's favorite fast dinner. After you have prepared and sliced all the ingredients, the dish requires only about 15 minutes of cooking. For a full meal serve with white rice (which takes about the same time to cook) and sliced fresh fruit. Sliced turkey breasts are a convenient and inexpensive substitute for the chicken breasts.

2 boneless chicken breasts	One 8-ounce package
3 tablespoons peanut oil	frozen Chinese pea pods
1 cup sliced celery	1 cup sliced fresh
1 small clove garlic,	mushrooms
minced	2 tablespoons cornstarch
One 14½-ounce can	3 to 4 tablespoons water
chicken broth	Salt to taste
2 tablespoons GF soy	¼ cup toasted slivered
sauce	almonds
1 tablespoon candied	
ginger, finely chopped	

Slice the chicken into long, thin strips. Using a wok or heavy frying pan, heat the oil, then add the chicken and sauté for 5 minutes. Stir in the celery and garlic and continue cooking for another 3 minutes.

Add the chicken broth, soy sauce, and ginger. Heat to boiling before adding the pea pods and mushrooms. Cover and simmer for 5 minutes (do not overcook).

Mix the cornstarch and the water. Stir into the chicken mixture and cook until the liquid thickens, 1 or 2 minutes. Taste and add salt if necessary (this will depend on the saltiness of the broth).

Pour the stir-fry onto a round serving platter immediately and top with the almonds. Serve rice separately. *Makes 4 servings.*

CASHEW CHICKEN

My favorite Chinese chicken dish. This recipe is from the Oregon State University Extension Service. The secret of easy stir-frying is to have everything cut and prepared before you heat your skillet. Then dinner is on the table in minutes. Serve with white rice, which you can begin cooking before you start the stir-fry. If you use a Teflon pan, you can reduce the amount of oil slightly.

2 chicken breasts, skinned and boned
3/4 cup cashew nuts
One 5-ounce can bamboo shoots, drained and sliced (optional)
8 fresh mushrooms, sliced
1 stalk celery, sliced on diagonal
One 6-ounce package frozen Chinese pea pods, thawed, or 15 fresh pea pods with strings removed, lightly sprinkled with salt
6 tablespoons vegetable oil, for frying

Marinade

1 tablespoon GF soy sauce
1 tablespoon cornstarch
1 tablespoon sherry
1 clove garlic, minced
1 teaspoon fresh gingerroot, grated
1/2 teaspoon salt

Sauce

3/4 cup water
1 tablespoon GF soy sauce
1 tablespoon cornstarch
1/2 teaspoon sugar

Wash the chicken and slice it into thin strips.
In a large bowl, combine all the marinade ingredients.
Add the chicken and let it sit for 15 minutes.
Measure the nuts and prepare the vegetables.
Sauce: In measuring cup combine sauce ingredients.
In a wok or large frying pan, heat 1 tablespoon of the oil over medium heat. Sauté the nuts until lightly browned. Remove to a large bowl.
In the same pan, heat 2 tablespoons of the oil on high heat. Add

the bamboo shoots (if used), mushrooms, and celery. Stir-fry for 2 minutes, or until the vegetables are crisp tender. Remove to the large bowl.

In the pan, heat 1 tablespoon of the oil on high. Add the pea pods and stir-fry for 1 minute. Remove to the bowl.

Heat the remaining 2 tablespoons oil on high. Add the marinated chicken and stir-fry for 4 minutes, or until meat is white. Return contents of bowl to pan. Stir the sauce and pour into the pan. Stir and cook until the sauce is thickened. *Makes 5 or 6 servings.*

TURKEY

STUFFED TURKEY ROLLS

A simple and tasty way of using the handy turkey slices now on the market. Topped with cranberry sauce, this make-ahead dish is a good family dinner or party casserole.

1¹/₄ cups soft GF bread
  crumbs
1 tablespoon minced onion
2 tablespoons minced
  celery
¹/₂ teaspoon poultry
  seasoning
Salt and pepper to taste
1 tablespoon chopped
  pecans (optional)
1 tablespoon butter or
  margarine, melted

¹/₄ cup (approximately)
  chicken broth
1¹/₂ pounds turkey breast
  slices (8 slices)

Sauce

One 4-ounce can jellied
  cranberry sauce
2 to 3 tablespoons water,
  for thinning

Preheat oven to 350°.

In a small bowl, combine the bread crumbs, onion, celery, poultry seasoning, salt and pepper, and pecans (if used). Pour in the butter.

Add enough of the chicken broth to make a dressing that just holds together.

Coat a 7" × 7" baking dish with vegetable oil spray. Salt and pepper the turkey slices (if desired). Onto each slice, spoon about 1 tablespoon of the dressing. Roll up and place, seam side down, in the baking dish, packing them tightly so they don't unroll during cooking.

Thin the cranberry sauce with 2 to 3 tablespoons water and pour over the rolls. Bake for about 1¼ hours, covering with aluminum foil for the first hour of baking time, until tender. *Makes 3 or 4 servings.*

TURKEY LOAF

A firm, well-seasoned meat loaf sure to win compliments. Good hot or cold, it slices well and makes great turkey sandwiches. Break it up and mix with mayonnaise and chopped pickles for stuffing pita bread. GF pickles can be found in some health food stores, or make your own (pages 252 and 253).

1½ pounds ground turkey (dark meat makes a moister loaf)	1 teaspoon Worcestershire sauce
¾ cup GF dry cereal, crushed	½ teaspoon thyme
	½ teaspoon marjoram
1 tablespoon GF soy sauce	½ teaspoon basil
1½ tablespoons butter or margarine, melted	1 teaspoon dried parsley
	1 egg, beaten slightly
	1 teaspoon salt, or to taste

Preheat oven to 350°.

In a large bowl, mix all the ingredients thoroughly. Shape the meat into a round loaf and place in a medium-size casserole. Bake, uncovered, for 1 hour. Let stand for about 10 minutes before slicing. *Makes 5 or 6 servings.*

MEDITERRANEAN MEATBALLS

I use ground turkey in this delightfully different recipe for meatballs, but you may substitute lamb. Double the recipe for a potluck or party.

1 1/4 pounds ground turkey
1/2 cup grated onion
1 egg, beaten
1 1/2 tablespoons chopped raisins
1 tablespoon chopped walnuts or pecans
1 tablespoon minced fresh parsley
Dash pepper

1/2 teaspoon salt, or to taste
1/2 teaspoon cinnamon
1/4 teaspoon allspice
1/4 teaspoon nutmeg
1 1/2 tablespoons margarine, melted
1 to 2 tablespoons vegetable oil, for frying

Preheat oven to 350°.

In a medium mixing bowl, knead together all the ingredients except the oil until well mixed and smooth. With wet hands, form the mixture into 1-inch balls.

In a frying pan, heat part of the oil. Fry about a third of the balls at a time on medium high, shaking the pan to keep the balls rounded and browning on all sides. Cook until brown all over. Drain on paper toweling and then put in a 2-quart casserole. Brown the remaining turkey balls in batches, using more oil if necessary.

When all the meatballs are browned, bake the casserole for 30 minutes to complete cooking. If you prefer, refrigerate the casserole to pull out and finish cooking just before serving. These are good both hot and cold. *Makes 4 or 5 servings.*

DRESSING AND SALSA

CRANBERRY DRESSING

An extraordinary accompaniment to chicken or pork, this slightly sweet, slightly tart dressing sparks up any meal. This recipe will stuff one roasting hen, but it can be cut to pack beside a pork roast or pieces of chicken, or doubled to stuff a 10- to 12-pound turkey.

4 cups GF bread, crumbled
1/2 cup fresh cranberries, chopped
1/3 cup pecans, chopped
1 1/2 tablespoons sugar
2 to 3 teaspoons grated orange rind
1/2 cup chicken stock or water

4 tablespoons (1/2 stick) margarine or butter
1 cup diced celery
3 to 4 green onions, sliced thin
1/2 teaspoon cinnamon
1/4 teaspoon cloves
Salt to taste

In a large mixing bowl, combine the bread, cranberries, pecans, sugar, and orange rind. Measure the chicken stock to be added later to desired consistency. (Breads absorb differently.)

In a medium frying pan, melt the margarine. Sauté the celery and onions seasoned with the cinnamon, cloves, and salt for about 3 minutes. Add to the bread mixture. Tumble and add the chicken stock, a little at a time, until desired consistency is reached. The meat juices will add moisture when the dressing is used as a stuffing. If baked outside the meat, the stuffing will dry some. *Makes 5 to 6 servings.*

CRANBERRY SALSA

Try this different cranberry sauce to serve with your turkey. It keeps so well it can be made several days ahead.

1 cup fresh or frozen
   cranberries
1/2 cup honey
1/4 cup toasted almonds or
   pine nuts
1/4 cup sour cream or
   nondairy substitute

1 teaspoon prepared
   horseradish
2 tablespoons chopped
   onion
3 tablespoons orange juice
1 tablespoon grated orange
   rind

Wash the cranberries. Toast the almonds or pine nuts in a 350° oven for 8 to 10 minutes, until lightly browned. Let cool.

Place all ingredients in a blender or food processor. Blend for 1 to 2 minutes. Refrigerate for several hours before serving. Keep refrigerated. *Makes approximately 1 1/2 cups salsa.*

SEAFOOD

FISH

Elegant Alaskan Halibut
Norwegian Fish Cake
    Casserole
Baked Fish Sticks
Sole Almondine with Mock
    Hollandaise Sauce

SHELLFISH

Crab-Broccoli Bake
Shrimp-Rice Pot
Coquilles Saint-Jacques

Indian Shrimp Cakes
Shrimp Curry
Deep Sea Delight
Tempura Batter for Seafood
Scalloped Oysters

SEE ALSO

Crab or Lobster Quiche
Norwegian Fish Balls
Fettuccine with Shrimp and
    Scallops
Egg Fu Yung

A dedicated seafood lover would probably be content to eat his or her fresh fish poached, broiled, steamed, or baked—with a squeeze of lemon, a sprinkle of seasoning, or a bit of tartar sauce or hollandaise sauce. Or he or she can choose, as many of our local seafood restaurants do, to marinate fish in a teriyaki sauce before barbecuing or grilling it. See page 301 for a simple marinade for chicken that is also tasty with seafood (the fish should not cook in the marinade).

Not everyone is a dedicated fish lover. Nor does everyone have access, as I do, to freshly harvested seafood. Still, you can enjoy air-freighted, flash frozen, canned, or imitation seafood in many recipes. For you, this chapter contains a few of my favorites, using seafood in dishes that are a bit more flavorful than simple poached fish.

I've included shrimp cakes and fish casseroles along with a wonderful Deep Sea Delight, which can use a variety of seafoods—fresh, canned, or imitation.

If you serve your guests—especially those who think they don't enjoy seafood—any of these, you could be surprised at the praise you'll receive.

FISH

ELEGANT ALASKAN HALIBUT

Although halibut is often dry, this tasty, moist, baked entrée from Alaska is not. It can be prepared ahead and put into the oven just 30 minutes before serving time.

1 1/2 pounds halibut
   fillets
Lemon pepper to
   taste
1/2 to 3/4 cup mayonnaise
Paprika

1/2 cup sliced almonds, 3
   to 4 tablespoons sliced
   green onions, or 1/2 to
   3/4 cup grated Cheddar
   cheese, for topping
   (optional)

Preheat oven to 350°.

Wash the halibut and slice all the fillets to an even 1/2-inch thickness. If possible, keep the pieces about 4 by 3 inches. Place them in a single layer covering the bottom of a greased baking dish. Sprinkle with lemon pepper. Cover with the mayonnaise to the thickness of cake frosting. Decorate with a scattering of paprika. If desired, halfway through baking, top with the Cheddar cheese. Bake for about 30 minutes, or until the fish flakes easily. For a dressier dish, scatter the top with the almonds or green onions. *Makes 4 to 5 servings.*

NORWEGIAN FISH CAKE
CASSEROLE

Absolutely wonderful! Fish cakes deep-fried, then baked in a tasty sauce are a little more trouble to make than baked fish, but well worth the effort, and they can be done ahead of time. The recipe can easily be doubled.

Fish Cakes

1¹/₂ pounds bottom fish (cod, halibut, or snapper)
1 small onion
1 egg
1¹/₂ tablespoons potato starch flour
¹/₄ teaspoon nutmeg
¹/₈ teaspoon mace
¹/₄ teaspoon pepper
³/₄ cup evaporated milk or fresh nondairy liquid

³/₄ teaspoon salt
Vegetable oil, for deep frying

Butter Sauce

¹/₄ cup (¹/₂ stick) butter or margarine
¹/₂ cup rice flour
2 cups chicken stock
3 green onions, sliced thin
1 teaspoon salt
¹/₄ teaspoon pepper

Wash and remove any bones or skin from the fish. Place the fish and onion in a food processor fitted with a metal blade and process until thoroughly pulped.

Place in a mixing bowl and, using an electric mixer, beat in the egg, flour, nutmeg, mace, and pepper. Gradually add the milk, beating until light and fluffy, about 15 minutes. Stir in the salt.

In a deep fat fryer or a deep heavy pan, heat 2 inches of the oil. Drop small egg-sized cakes of batter from a wet spoon into the oil. Cook the cakes until brown and crusty. Drain on paper toweling while making the sauce.

Preheat oven to 350°.

Butter Sauce: In a 1¹/₂-quart saucepan, melt the butter and add the flour. Slowly add the chicken stock, stirring constantly. Add the green onion, salt, and pepper. Cook over medium heat until thickened.

Place the fish cakes in a 2-quart casserole. Pour the sauce over them and bake for 45 minutes. (If making ahead, refrigerate the fish cakes and sauce; bring to room temperature before baking.) *Makes 4 or 5 servings.*

BAKED FISH STICKS

A great-tasting fish dish, easy to prepare and only a few minutes' time in the oven. Use any firm, mild fish such as snapper, cod, halibut, or other. If possible, purchase thick fillets, for they cut into the best sticks.

> **2 pounds firm, mild fish**
> **2 cups crushed corn chips**
> **1 teaspoon seafood seasoning**
> **1 cup plain yogurt**

Preheat oven to 350°.

Wash and cut the fish into 1-by-4-inch strips.

Crush the corn chips to a fine breading. Add the seasoning. Place in a low, flat pan or on a sheet of aluminum foil.

Pour the yogurt into a flat bowl. Roll the fish in the yogurt, then in the corn chips. Place in a greased 9″ × 13″ pan or cookie sheet with at least a half inch between sticks. Bake for 20 to 25 minutes, or until the fish flakes easily and the crust is brown. Serve immediately. *Makes 4 or 5 servings.*

SOLE ALMONDINE
with Mock Hollandaise Sauce

One of my favorite fish dishes can't be ordered in a restaurant because the sole is usually rolled in flour before being dipped in the egg. You can buy some GF dry hollandaise sauce mixes, but I recommend this mock hollandaise recipe for an easy, tasty sauce that cooks the egg yolks and never curdles. Any leftover keeps well in the refrigerator to reheat and serve over broccoli, cauliflower, or carrots at another meal. With this fish I like to serve a fresh cabbage slaw and little red potatoes cooked in their skins and topped with parsley.

1¹/₂ **pounds sole fillets**
Salt and pepper to taste
1 egg, beaten slightly
**1 tablespoon vegetable oil,
   for frying**
¹/₃ **cup sliced almonds, for
   topping**

Mock Hollandaise Sauce

2 egg yolks
1 cup mayonnaise
2 teaspoons lemon juice
**2 tablespoons butter or
   margarine**

Wash and cut the fish into 4-inch sections. Add salt and pepper.

In a large frying pan or griddle, heat the oil. Dip the fish in the egg and fry quickly, turning when first side is lightly browned and fish is white. When done, divide among 4 serving plates. Top with 1 to 2 tablespoons Mock Hollandaise Sauce and a sprinkling of almonds. Serve immediately. *Makes 4 servings.*

Sauce: If making this Hollandaise, do before cooking the fish and keep it warm until ready to serve. Beat the egg yolks in a blender until very light and thick. Add the mayonnaise, a quarter cup at a time, beating until very stiff. Add the lemon juice. Transfer to the top of a double boiler over hot (but not boiling) water. Cook, adding the butter, beating constantly with a slotted spoon or wire whip until the eggs have further thickened the sauce and it is very smooth. If too thick, add 1 to 3 tablespoons of hot water, 1 at a time. *Makes 1¹/₃ cups.*

SHELLFISH

CRAB-BROCCOLI BAKE

Serve this delicious main-dish seafood-vegetable casserole with slices of fresh fruit. Add some GF bread or a roll and you have dinner. For two to three servings, halve the recipe and use a 1¹/₂-quart baking dish.

¹/₂ pound (2 cups) fresh
  crabmeat or two 6-ounce
  cans crabmeat
4 cups broccoli florets or
  two 10-ounce packages
  frozen broccoli
4 tablespoons butter
¹/₄ cup chopped onion

1 teaspoon salt
4 tablespoons rice flour
2 cups milk or nondairy
  liquid
2 cups grated Cheddar
  cheese
2 tablespoons lemon juice

Preheat oven to 350°.

Pick over the crabmeat to be sure there are no shells, or open and drain the cans. Set aside.

Cook the broccoli until it is just barely tender. Drain and place it in a 2-quart casserole.

In a heavy saucepan, melt the butter and sauté the onion until clear. Stir in the salt and flour. Add the milk slowly, stirring continually. Turn heat to medium and cook until thickened. Add the cheese and stir until melted. Add the lemon juice and the crabmeat. Spoon the cheese-crab sauce over the broccoli. Bake for 30 minutes. *Makes 5 or 6 servings.*

SHRIMP-RICE POT

This tasty French-inspired dish may have originally featured freshwater crayfish, but flash frozen shrimp is now available in most fish markets, so one need not wade the creeks for the crayfish. Serve a salad or fruit slices with this easy-to-make dish for a full meal.

1 pound uncooked shrimp	2 cups hot chicken broth
1 cup frozen baby peas	$1/4$ cup dry white wine or
2 tablespoons margarine or	$1/4$ cup water plus
butter	1 tablespoon lemon juice
$3/4$ cup sliced green onions	1 teaspoon salt, or to taste
2 cloves garlic, minced	if broth is salted
1 cup white rice	

Wash the shrimp and cut them into $1/2$-inch sections. Put aside. Measure the peas and let thaw.

In a heavy 2-quart saucepan, melt the margarine. Add the green onions and garlic. Sauté over medium heat until the onions are clear. Stir in the rice and sauté on low heat for about 2 minutes.

Add the hot chicken broth and wine and bring to a boil. Reduce heat to low, cover, and cook for 10 minutes. Add the shrimp and the peas, stirring them in gently. Cover and cook until the shrimp, peas, and rice are done, 5 to 10 minutes. Season to taste with salt, if necessary. Serve immediately. *Makes 4 servings.*

COQUILLES SAINT-JACQUES

No seafood lover should miss these delicious scallops. Their mild, delicate flavor is enhanced by the simple seasonings and wine. Serve with a tossed salad or sliced fruit and crusty bread for a full meal. For a hungry family, add a brown rice pilaf.

1 pint scallops	1/4 cup water
3 tablespoons butter or margarine	1 teaspoon chopped parsley
1 shallot or 2 green onions	Salt and pepper to taste
1 tablespoon butter or margarine, divided	1/4 cup GF bread crumbs
1 tablespoon rice flour	2 tablespoons grated Parmesan cheese
1/2 cup white wine	

Slice the scallops to about 1/4 inch thick. Chop the shallot or slice the green onions (using some of the green part).

In a large skillet, heat the butter. Sauté the scallop slices with the shallot for about 3 minutes. Stir in the flour, add the wine and the water, and simmer for about 10 more minutes, or until the sauce is slightly reduced and thickened. Add the parsley and season with the salt and pepper, if necessary.

Fill 4 small baking dishes or shells with the mixture. Sprinkle with the bread crumbs and the cheese. Dot with the remaining 1 tablespoon butter and place under the broiler to brown lightly. *Makes 4 servings.*

INDIAN SHRIMP CAKES

These delicious spiced patties combine a small amount of shrimp with inexpensive white fish for a tasty seafood main dish. Serve with coleslaw and a fresh muffin for a full meal.

12 ounces white fish (cod, snapper, sole, or halibut)
6 ounces cooked shrimp, chopped
4 green onions, chopped
1 tablespoon grated fresh gingerroot
2 tablespoons chopped fresh parsley
2 cups fresh GF bread crumbs, divided
Salt and cayenne pepper to taste
1 egg yolk, beaten
2 tablespoons lemon juice
1/4 cup rice flour
1/2 cup soy flour
1 tablespoon ground coriander
1/2 cup water
1/4 cup oil

Wash the fish and pat dry with paper toweling. Remove any bones and skin.

Mince the fish and place it in a medium mixing bowl. Add the shrimp, green onions, grated gingerroot, parsley, 1/2 cup of the bread crumbs, and the salt and cayenne. Mix in the egg yolk and lemon juice. Form into sixteen 1/2-inch-thick patties. Roll these in the remaining bread crumbs to coat completely.

In a small flat-bottomed bowl, make a batter of the rice flour, soy flour, coriander, salt and cayenne to taste, and the water. Beat until smooth.

In a large skillet, heat the oil. Dip patties in the batter and fry for 2 to 3 minutes on each side, or until brown. Drain on paper toweling and serve immediately. *Makes 4 or 5 servings.*

SHRIMP CURRY

A mild, sweet curry, easy to make. If you've shied away from the heavily spiced curries of India, try this Indonesian dish. Serve it with white rice and fruit slices or a cool green salad.

4 tablespoons (1/2 stick)
  margarine or butter
3 tablespoons chopped
  onion
1 clove garlic, minced
2 tablespoons rice flour
1/2 teaspoon salt
1 tablespoon sugar
1 tablespoon curry powder
1 teaspoon grated fresh
  gingerroot

2 cups chicken broth
1 to 2 cups cooked shrimp
1/2 cup sour cream or
  nondairy substitute
1/2 cup chopped peanuts
  (optional)
2 green onions, chopped
  (optional)

In a large frying pan, melt the margarine. Add the onion and garlic and sauté until tender.

Mix together the flour, salt, sugar, curry powder, and gingerroot. Stir into the frying pan. Cook for 1 minute or 2, then add the chicken broth and bring to a simmer until thickened. Allow to cook on low heat for a short time, until the flavors blend. Stir in the shrimp, turn down the heat, and cook until the shrimp are heated through. At the last minute, add the sour cream; heat for a few seconds before removing from the stove.

Serve over rice on individual serving plates, topped with the peanuts and green onions, if desired. *Makes 4 servings.*

DEEP SEA DELIGHT

This casserole can be a real delight for the cook and for the ones to whom this is served. Alter it by using a variety of seafoods or by exchanging the cooked noodles for 1¹/₂ cups GF bread cubes. Prepare it about 45 minutes before serving, or hours ahead. Serve with a salad for a full meal.

¹/₂ batch fresh egg noodles (page 228) or 6 ounces GF fettuccine

¹/₂ pound cooked crabmeat or lobster (fresh or GF imitation sirimi) or one 6¹/₂-ounce can tunafish

1 pound asparagus or one 15-ounce can cut asparagus

1 cup fresh sliced mushrooms or one 4-ounce can mushrooms

3 green onions, sliced thin

¹/₂ teaspoon salt

¹/₈ teaspoon pepper

1 cup grated Cheddar cheese, divided

Sauce

2 tablespoons butter or margarine

2 tablespoons rice flour

¹/₂ teaspoon coriander

2 cups milk or nondairy liquid

2 tablespoons sherry

Preheat oven to 350°.

Cook the noodles in boiling salted water to which 1 tablespoon of oil has been added until al dente. Drain.

Drain the tunafish, if used.

Cook the fresh asparagus for 5 minutes or drain the canned. Drain the canned mushrooms (if used).

Sauce: In a medium saucepan, melt the butter. Blend in the flour and coriander. Add the milk, stirring constantly. Cook until thickened slightly. Add the sherry and remove from heat.

Grease a 2¹/₂-quart casserole. Add, in order, the noodles, crabmeat, asparagus, mushrooms, green onions, salt, pepper, and ³/₄ cup of the cheese. Pour on the sauce and mix slightly. Top with the remaining ¹/₄ cup cheese. (If prepared early in the day and refrigerated, cool the sauce before adding to the casserole.) Bake for 35 to 40 minutes, or slightly longer if the dish has been taken from the refrigerator. *Makes 6 servings.*

TEMPURA BATTER FOR SEAFOOD

If you've been craving the deep-fried fish of "fish and chips," look no further. This light, delicate batter is tasty on all seafood. Do as the Japanese do and cut your fish into bite-sized pieces to enjoy more of the batter and save time in cooking. Use any firm white fish: halibut, cod, snapper, or other. Try this also with shrimp, oysters, or scallops.

2 cups fish or other seafood	1/4 teaspoon xanthan gum
1 egg, beaten	1 teaspoon seafood seasoning
1 cup Fresca, 7UP, or Sprite	Salt to taste, if necessary
1/4 cup cornstarch	1/2 teaspoon baking powder
1/2 cup rice flour (sweet rice best)	3 cups vegetable oil, for deep frying

Wash and cut fish into cubes. If using shrimp, slit them partially through lengthwise, leaving the tail on. For oysters, drain and cut large ones in half.

In a medium bowl, beat the egg. Add the Fresca.

Mix together the cornstarch, sweet rice flour, xanthan gum, seafood seasoning, salt, and baking powder. Beat half the flour mixture into the egg, then stir in the rest. Batter a few pieces of fish at a time, then let drain.

In an automatic frying kettle or frying pan, heat the oil to 375°. Gently drop in the battered and drained fish, cooking only a few pieces at a time. Turn once as they brown. Remove and drain on paper toweling. Serve while hot. *Makes 4 servings.*

NOTE: If you are cooking fish and vegetables at the same time, use the Tempura Batter for Vegetables (page 249) for both.

SCALLOPED OYSTERS

This was a Christmas Eve dish in our Northwestern family. With fresh shucked oysters now available in the nearest supermarket, it can be a tasty gourmet dish anytime, even for those living far from the sea.

1 pint fresh small to
   medium oysters with
   liquor
$^1/_2$ cup GF bread crumbs
1 cup Weight Watchers
   Harvest Rice Crispbread,
   crushed (see Note)

$^1/_4$ cup ($^1/_2$ stick) butter or
   margarine, melted
2 tablespoons cream or
   nondairy substitute
$^1/_2$ teaspoon lemon pepper

Preheat oven to 350°.

Drain the oysters, reserving $^1/_4$ cup of the liquor. Set aside.

In a medium bowl, mix the bread crumbs and Crispbread. Stir in the melted butter.

In a measuring cup, combine the cream and lemon pepper with the oyster liquor.

Place one-third of the bread crumb mixture in an 8″ × 8″ baking dish. Add half the oysters, then pour in half of the liquid. Add another third of the crumbs, then the rest of the oysters and liquid. Top with the remaining crumbs. Bake for about 30 minutes. *Serves 6.*

NOTE: The suggested cracker contains soy. If you are allergic to soy, substitute $^3/_4$ cup GF bread crumbs.

Time-saving Mixes

BAKING MIXES

Triple-Duty Muffin
    Mix
Buttermilk Pancake
    Mix
Mary G's Biscuit
    Mix

DRY SOUPS

Creamed Soup Base
Onion Soup Mix

BREADING

GF Seasoned Breading

Most packaged mixes, whether for soup, seasoning, or baking, contain gluten in some form. This means we must start from scratch each time we prepare a dish—definitely a frustrating and time-consuming prospect to the already overworked cook.

At the prodding of another celiac, I've developed a few seasoning formulas, powdered soups, and baking mixes. The seasoning and soup mixes are time-savers at home; the baking mixes are lifesavers when traveling.

I remember early in my life as a celiac visiting friends halfway across the country, and feeling such pangs of jealousy when watching others eat the muffins that I'd had to refuse that I swore it would never happen again. After that, I packed fewer clothes and took some of my own goodies, although they often grew stale by the end of a trip. Now I've solved the problem of fresh GF baking with these prepared mixes. Carry them along when visiting relatives or friends. Take plenty, for they're so good you'll want to share.

For the GF flour mix used in some of the baking mixes:

> Blend together: 2 parts white rice flour
> 2/3 part potato starch flour
> 1/3 part tapioca flour

If you don't want to mix your own, there are a few dry mixes for some soups, dips, and sauces, but they are not always available on the grocery shelves *and they sometimes change formulas, so always read labels.* You'll also find some packaged baking mixes sold in health food stores and by mail order (see "Where to Find Gluten-free Products," page 343).

BAKING MIXES

TRIPLE-DUTY MUFFIN MIX

This mix makes great muffins, a quick cake, or even tops fruit for a cobbler. Use it at home or carry it when you travel. See the variations for the many ways to vary the taste.

2¼ cups rice flour	1 tablespoon Egg Replacer
½ cup potato starch flour	1 teaspoon xanthan gum
½ cup tapioca flour	⅓ cup sugar
1 teaspoon baking soda	2 teaspoons dried lemon
4 teaspoons baking powder	peel or powdered vanilla
1 teaspoon salt	

Mix together all the ingredients and store in an airtight container. *Makes enough for 4 batches of baking.*

TO MAKE MUFFINS: To 1 cup of mix, beat together 2 eggs, 2 tablespoons vegetable oil or melted butter, and ⅓ cup liquid (buttermilk, milk, nondairy liquid, fruit juice, or carbonated drink). Pour into the flour mix and beat until smooth. Do not overbeat. Spoon into 6 greased muffin cups and bake in a preheated 375° oven for 12 to 15 minutes. *Makes 6 muffins.*

TO VARY TASTE: You may add ¼ cup raisins, nuts, mashed bananas or kiwifruit, chopped dates, or ⅓ cup grated fresh apple.

TO MAKE COBBLER: Mix as for muffins and drop the mix by spoonfuls atop 1 quart of fresh berries or sliced peaches (which have been heated with sufficient sugar to sweeten in 1¹/2 cups water) in an 8″ × 8″ pan. Bake in a preheated 350° oven for 20 to 25 minutes, or until the top is brown and springs back when lightly pressed.

To Make an 8-Inch Single-layer Round Cake: Mix as for muffins but add 1 more tablespoon sugar to 1 cup mix and spoon dough into a greased pan. Bake in a preheated 350° oven for 20 to 25 minutes. Serve with whipped cream and fruit, or frost to your taste.

BUTTERMILK PANCAKE MIX

How easy to reach for the prepared mix, add fresh egg, water, and oil, and have your pancakes ready to go in seconds!

4 cups GF flour mix	2 teaspoons baking soda
1 cup buttermilk powder	4 teaspoons Egg Replacer
¹/4 cup sugar	(optional)
4 teaspoons baking powder	

Combine the ingredients and mix well. Store in an airtight container on the pantry shelf. *Makes 4 batches of pancakes (see below).*
Beat together:

2 eggs
1 cup water
2 tablespoons oil

Pancakes: Place 1¹/3 cups of the dry mix in a bowl. Add the egg mixture and beat until smooth. Do not overbeat.
Drop spoonfuls of the batter onto a hot greased griddle and cook until top is full of tiny bubbles and the underside is brown. Flip and brown the other side. *Makes ten 4-inch pancakes.*

MARY G'S BISCUIT MIX

One of my readers suggested this mix she modified from my original biscuit recipe in The Gluten-free Gourmet. *For traveling, she makes the full recipe and separates it into four plastic packets with complete mixing and baking directions on the bag. Store in a cool place or refrigerate until needed.*

4 tablespoons sugar	8 teaspoons baking powder
2 cups rice flour	2 teaspoons baking soda
1¹/₃ cups potato starch flour	2 teaspoons salt
	³/₄ cup shortening

In a large bowl, mix together all the dry ingredients. Cut in the shortening until the mixture is crumbly. *Makes 4 batches of biscuits.*

TO MAKE BISCUITS: Add 1 beaten egg and ¹/₃ cup buttermilk to a quarter of the mixture. Stir gently to moisten. Roll out onto a rice-floured board and cut into biscuit shapes, or drop by spoonfuls onto a greased baking sheet.

Bake in a preheated oven at 400° for 12 to 15 minutes. *Makes 8 to 10 biscuits.*

TO TOP COOKED STEWS OR CHICKEN PIES: Make as for biscuits and place the dough on the prepared meat dishes in casseroles. Bake in a preheated 350° oven for 20 to 25 minutes or until the biscuits are done.

DRY SOUPS

CREAMED SOUP BASE

Use this when a recipe calls for one can of creamed soup. A few table-spoons of this plus water will yield the equivalent of a can of chicken soup. See below for the various ways to use the base.

1 cup noninstant dry milk or nondairy substitute	1/2 teaspoon pepper
1 cup white rice flour	1/2 teaspoon salt
2 tablespoons dried minced onions	3 tablespoons GF powdered chicken soup base

Combine and mix well. Store in an airtight container on pantry shelf. *This will make the equivalent of 6 cans of soup.*

To Make the Soup: Blend 3 to 4 tablespoons (3 for thin soup; 4 for thick) of the dry mix with 1/4 cup cold water. Add 1 cup hot or cold water and cook, stirring, until the soup thickens.

For a Tasty Cream Sauce: Melt 1 tablespoon butter or margarine in a pan and add 1 teaspoon chopped chives before adding soup base. Add 1 cup hot water and cook as above.

To Use in Casserole Dishes: If a recipe (such as scalloped potatoes, etc.) calls for canned soup and is to be baked for more than 1 hour, tumble 3 to 4 tablespoons of the above mix with the other ingredients and pour on 1 1/4 to 1 1/2 cups hot water.

Cream of Mushroom Soup: Follow directions to make soup, but use liquid from one 4-ounce can of sliced mushrooms as part of the water and, after the soup thickens, add the mushrooms.

CREAM OF TOMATO SOUP: Follow directions for soup, using one 5.5-ounce can of V-8 juice as part of the liquid.

NOTE: For the lactose intolerant, try using the powdered baby formulas Isomil (soy) or Pregestimil (corn), instead of Lacto-free nondairy dry powder, for the best flavor.

ONION SOUP MIX

Easy to make and better tasting than a purchased packet, which is often high in sodium and MSG. Use this mix for dips, for seasoning meats, casseroles and stews, and in Pink Onion Bread (page 66). When a recipe calls for a packet of dried onion soup, use two tablespoons of the mix, increasing or decreasing to taste.

1/2 teaspoon onion powder	1 tablespoon vegetable oil
1/2 teaspoon onion salt	1/2 cup minced dehydrated
1/4 teaspoon sugar	onions
1/4 teaspoon Kitchen	1 tablespoon potato starch
Bouquet Browning Sauce	flour

In a small bowl, combine the onion powder, onion salt, and sugar. Add the Kitchen Bouquet Sauce and oil. Stir until seasonings are uniformly colored.

Add the dehydrated onion and mix thoroughly until an even color is achieved, which may take several minutes. Stir in the potato starch flour to keep flakes separated. Store in an airtight container on a kitchen shelf. *Makes 1/2 cup mix.*

DIP: Add 2 rounded tablespoons to each cup of sour cream or sour cream substitute. Let stand for 24 hours for flavors to meld.

POT ROAST: Season with 1 to 2 tablespoons of mix according to taste.

BREADING

GF SEASONED BREADING

Missing that handy Shake 'n Bake (full of gluten) for the pork chop, chicken, or fish? This mix can take its place. Make up this large batch and use for four or five meals.

2 cups GF bread crumbs, dry
1/4 cup cornstarch
1 tablespoon paprika, or to taste
4 teaspoons salt
2 teaspoons sugar
2 teaspoons onion powder
2 teaspoons oregano
1/2 teaspoon garlic powder
1/2 teaspoon cumin
1/4 cup vegetable shortening

In a food processor, whirl the bread crumbs until fine. Mix with the cornstarch, paprika, salt, sugar, onion powder, oregano, garlic powder, and cumin. Cut in the shortening until the mixture is crumbly. Store in a covered container in a cool, dry place.

To use, dip the fish, chicken, or chops into milk, nondairy liquid, or yogurt and then into the coating. Place in a single layer in an ungreased baking dish. Bake fish at 400° for about 10 minutes, or until tender and flaky. Bake chicken at 350° for 45 to 50 minutes. Bake chops at 325° for 1 hour. *Makes about 3 cups breading.*

THE GLUTEN-FREE
DIET

A diet free of the toxic gluten protein found in wheat, rye, barley, and oats.

The following list was compiled from information supplied by my physician, the Gluten Intolerance Group of North America, the Celiac Disease Foundation, and the Canadian Celiac Association. I followed the standards of the United States organizations.

Please note food regulations vary from country to country. For example, in Canada whiskey is on the allowed list, and so are condiments and pickles with distilled vinegar (not so in the United States). In the United Kingdom wheat starch is allowed, but it is not in either the United States or Canada.

Foods Allowed	Foods to Avoid
BEVERAGES	
Coffee, tea, carbonated beverages, cocoa (Bakers, Hershey's, Nestlé), rum, tequila, vodka (if made from potatoes or grapes), wine.	Postum, Ovaltine, beer, ale, gin, vodka (if made from grain), whiskey, some flavored coffees, some herbal teas.

Foods Allowed	Foods to Avoid

BREADS

Breads made with gluten-free flours only (rice, potato starch, soy, tapioca, corn) either baked at home or purchased from companies that produce GF products. Rice crackers or cakes, corn tortillas.	All breads made with wheat, oats, rye, barley flours. All purchased crackers, croutons, bread crumbs, wafers, biscuits, and doughnuts containing any gluten flours. Graham, soda, and snack crackers, tortillas containing wheat.

CEREALS

Cornmeal, hot rice cereals, hominy grits, gluten-free cold rice, and corn cereals (those without malt).	All cereals containing wheat, rye, oats, or barley (both as the grain and in the flavoring, such as malt flavoring, malt syrup).

DAIRY PRODUCTS

Milk (fresh, dry, evaporated, or condensed), buttermilk, cream, sour cream, butter, cheese (except those that contain oat gum), whipped cream, yogurt (plain and flavored if GF), ice cream (if GF), artificial cream (if GF).	Malted milk, artificial cream (if not GF), some chocolate milk drinks, some commercial ice creams, some processed cheese spreads, flavored yogurt (containing gluten).

DESSERTS

Any pie, cake, cookie, or other desserts made with GF flours and flavorings, gelatins, custards, homemade puddings (rice, cornstarch, tapioca).	All pies, cakes, cookies, etc. that contain any wheat, oat, rye, or barley flour or flavoring, most commercial pudding mixes, ice cream cones, prepared cake mixes.

Foods Allowed	Foods to Avoid

FATS

Margarine, vegetable oil, nuts, GF mayonnaise, shortening, lard, some salad dressings.	Some commercial salad dressings, some mayonnaise.

FLOURS

Rice flour (brown and white), soy flour, potato starch flour, potato flour, tapioca flour, corn flour, cornmeal, cornstarch, rice bran, rice polish, arrowroot, nut or legume flours.	All flours or baking mixes containing wheat, rye, barley, or oats.

FRUITS AND JUICES

All fruit, fresh, frozen, canned (if GF), and dried (if not dusted with flour to prevent sticking).	Any commercially canned fruit with gluten thickening.

MEAT, FISH, POULTRY, AND EGGS

Any eggs (plain or in cooking), all fresh meats, poultry, fish and seafood, fish canned in oil, vegetable broth, or brine, GF prepared meats such as luncheon meats, tofu, GF imitation seafood.	Eggs in gluten-based sauce; imitation seafood containing gluten flour; prepared meats such as salami, frankfurters, etc. that contain gluten; some fish canned in HVP; self-basting turkeys injected with HVP.

PASTAS

GF homemade noodles, spaghetti, or other pasta, oriental rice noodles, bean threads, purchased GF pasta made with corn, rice, tapioca, and potato flours.	Noodles, spaghetti, macaroni, or other pasta made with gluten flours. Any canned pasta product.

Foods Allowed	Foods to Avoid

SOUPS AND CHOWDERS

Homemade broth and soups made with GF ingredients, some canned soups, some powdered soup bases, some GF dehydrated soups.	Most canned soups, most dehydrated soup mixes, bouillon and bouillon cubes containing HVP.

VEGETABLES

All plain fresh, frozen, or canned vegetables, dried peas, beans, and lentils.	All creamed, breaded, and escalloped vegetables, some canned baked beans, some prepared salad mixes.

SWEETS

Jellies, jams, honey, sugar, molasses, corn syrup, syrup, some commercial candies.	Some commercial candy, some cake decorations. Note: Icing sugar in Canada may contain wheat.

CONDIMENTS

Salt, pepper, herbs, food coloring, pure spices, rice, cider and wine vinegar, GF soy sauce, GF curry powder, baking powder, baking soda.	Some curry powder, some mixed spices, distilled vinegar (see Note on page 14), some ketchup, some prepared mustards, most soy sauces.

This is just a general list for your information. Always remember to read the full ingredient list when purchasing any product that might contain any form of gluten.

WHERE TO FIND GLUTEN-FREE PRODUCTS

When I wrote *The Gluten-free Gourmet* a decade ago, the suppliers for products without gluten were very few and the products they carried were very limited. That has changed and today there are over fifty large suppliers and a variety of gluten-free products are carried in health food stores and specialty markets. Many support groups sell the flours, mixes, and xanthan gum at their meetings or by mail order; otherwise you will find anything you need to bake with available from the list of suppliers below.

Even more exciting is the fact that in the last year or so, cake and bread mixes have joined the gluten-free cookies and crackers on a few grocery shelves and Asian stores have begun to carry fine white rice, tapioca, and potato starch flours. Mail-order suppliers have branched out into more than just cookies and mixes—some furnish main dishes either frozen or freeze dried to eat at home or when camping, others provide ready baked desserts.

With these many suppliers specializing in gluten-free goods, you should find all your baking needs close to home. But there are still a few flours (the Garfava and sorghum flours) featured in this revised edition that are so unusual they haven't reached regular markets, and these will have to be special ordered until health food stores carry them on a regular basis.

Alpineaire Foods (freeze-dried soups and meals for camping, hiking, and backpacking), 4031 Alvis Court, Rocklin, CA 95677; phone (800) 322-6325 or (916) 824-5000. Accepts orders by mail, phone, or fax. Some products can be found in sporting goods stores. Write or phone for a full product list.

Authentic Foods (baking mixes for pancakes, bread, and cakes; Garfava flour; brown and white rice flour; tapioca starch; potato flour and potato starch; xanthan gum; maple sugar; vanilla powder; rye flavor powder), 1850 West 169th Street, Suite B, Gardena CA 90247; phone (800) 806-4737 or (310) 366-7612, fax (310) 366-6938. Accepts orders by phone, mail, or fax. Write for complete product list. Some products can be found in health food stores.

Bob's Red Mill Natural Foods (wheat-free biscuit and baking mix, xanthan and guar gum, wheat-free flours, legume flours), 5209 SE International Way, Milwaukie, OR 97222; phone (800) 553-2258, fax (503) 653-1339. Web site: www.bobsredmill.com. Takes orders by mail, phone, or fax. Write for an order form. Some products can be found in health food stores and in health sections of grocery stores.

Cybros, Inc. (white rice flour and tapioca flour), PO Box 851, Waukesha, WI 53187-0851; phone (800) 876-2253. Accepts orders by mail or phone. Products can also be found in health food stores.

Dietary Specialties, Inc., a MenuDirect Company (crackers, baking mixes, prepared entrees, breads, snacks, pretzels, xanthan and guar gum, flavorings, dough enhancer), 865 Centennial Avenue, Piscataway, NJ 08854; phone (888) 636-MENU. Accepts orders by phone or mail or e-mail www.dietspec.com. Write or phone for list of products.

El Peto Products Ltd. (strictly gluten-free manufacturer and distributor of fresh-baked products, baking mixes, soups, pastas, gluten-free flours, cookbooks, snacks, and crackers; bean, rice, quinoa, millet, and other gluten-free flours milled specially for The Mill Stone), 41 Shoemaker Street, Kitchener, Ontario N2E 3G9, Canada; phone (800) 387-4064, fax (519) 743-8096, e-mail elpeto@golden.net, www.elpeto.com. Order by phone, fax, mail or e-mail. Some products can be found in specialty markets and health food stores.

Ener-G-Foods, Inc. (breads, rolls, buns, pizza shells, doughnuts, cookies, granola, and bars; xanthan gum; methocel; dough enhancer; almond meal; tapioca, bean, rice, and other gluten-free flours; and Bette Hagman's flour mixes, Egg Replacer, Lacto-Free, and cookbooks), PO Box 84487, Seattle, WA 98124; phone (800) 331-5222, fax (206) 764-3398. Accepts orders by phone, mail, fax, or secure Web site: www.ener-g.com. Phone for a catalog. Products can be found in some health food stores and specialty markets.

Food for Life Baking Co., Inc. (baked bread and muffins, pastas) PO Box 1434, Corona, CA 91718-1434; phone (800) 797-5090, fax (909) 279-1784. Takes orders by mail. Write for their order form. Products can be found in frozen-food section of specialty and natural food stores under Food for Life brand.

The Food Merchants (polenta and polenta pastas), 7120 W 117th Avenue B-1, Broomfield, CO 80020; phone (303) 404-2691, fax (303) 469-9630. Accepts orders by mail. Some products can be found in health food stores and some groceries. Phone for product list.

G1 Foods (cookies, breakfast bars, granola), 3536 17th Street, San Francisco, CA 94110; phone (415) 255-2139, fax (415) 863-3359. Accepts orders by mail, phone and fax. Write or phone for the order form.

The Gluten-Free Pantry, Inc. (gluten-free mixes, crackers, cookies, pastas, soups and baking supplies such as xanthan gum, guar gum, dough enhancer; a long list of gluten-free flours including white, brown and wild rice, garbanzo bean, several corn flours, and more), PO Box 840, Glastonbury, CT 06033; phone (800) 291-8386 or (860) 633-3826, fax (860) 633-6853, Web site www.glutenfree.com. Write or phone for their free catalog. Accepts orders by phone, mail, or fax.

Glutino.com (De-Ro-Ma) (breads, bagels, pizzas, cookies, mixes, pastas, baked items, and gluten-free flours), 1118 Berlier, Laval, Quebec H7L 3R9, Canada; phone (450) 629-7689 or (800) 363-3438 (DIET), fax (450) 629-4781. Call, fax or write for their catalog. Many items can be found in health food and grocery stores. Also sold through celiac organizations. Web site www.glutino.com.

Grain Process Enterprises, Ltd. (Romano, navy, and garbanzo bean flour; yellow pea flour; and other gluten-free flours including rice, buckwheat, millet, tapioca, potato and arrowroot; xanthan and guar gums), 115 Commander Blvd., Scarborough, Ontario M1S 3M7, Canada; phone (416) 291-3226, fax (416) 291-2159. Write or phone for their list. Takes orders by mail, phone, or fax. Some products can be found in health food stores.

Jowar Foods (sorghum flour), PO Box 775, Vega TX 79092; phone (806) 267-0820, fax (806) 267-0769. Accepts orders by phone, mail, or fax. Sorghum flour can be found in some health food stores and specialty markets.

The King Arthur Flour Co., INC. (rice and tapioca flours, potato starch, xanthan gum), PO Box 876, Norwich, VT 05055; phone (800) 827-6836, fax (800) 343-3002. Accepts orders by phone, fax, or mail. Please request a free King Arthur Flour Baker's Catalog.

Kinnikinnick Foods (breads; buns; bagels; doughnuts; cookies; pizza crusts; muffins; xanthan gum; guar gum; rice, corn, potato, bean and soya flours; other baking supplies), 10306-112 Street, Edmonton, Alberta T5K 1N1, Canada; phone (877) 503-4466, fax (780) 421-0456, toll free (877) 503-4466, e-mail info@kinnikinnick.com, Web site www.kinikinnick.com. Accepts orders via phone, mail, fax, secure Web site. Offers home delivery of all products to most areas in North America. Some products may be found in health food stores and some in regular grocery stores in the alternative foods section.

Mrs. Leeper's Pasta (gluten-free corn and rice pastas), 12455 Kerran Street, #200, Poway, CA 92064; phone (858) 486-1101, fax (858) 406-1770. Sold through health food stores and some gourmet sections in large grocery stores under the label Mrs. Leeper's Pasta or Michelle's Natural. Write or phone to inquire where distributed in your area. Mail orders will be filled for those who live too far from stores handling these products.

Legumes Plus, Inc. (lentil soups, chili, casserole and salad mixes), PO Box 383, Fairfield, WA 99012; phone (800) 845-1349, fax (509) 283-2314. Accepts orders by phone, mail, or fax. Some products can be found in health food and gourmet stores and specialty supermarkets.

Mendocino Gluten-free Products, Inc. (bread mix, pancake and waffle mix, general purpose flour), PO Box 277, Willits, CA 95490-0277;

phone (800) 297-5399, fax (707) 459-1834. Products marketed under Sylvan Border Farm label. Orders taken by phone, mail, or fax. Write or phone for an order form. Some products may be found in health food and grocery stores.

Nancy's Natural Foods (long list of gluten-free flours including sorghum and bean, xanthan gum, guar gum, milk powders and substitutes), 266 NW First Avenue, Suite A, Canby, OR 97013; phone (503) 266-3306, fax (503) 266-3306, e-mail nnfoods@juno.com. Accepts orders by phone, mail, and e-mail. Ask for their long list of gluten-free baking supplies.

Pamela's Products, Inc. (cookies, biscotti, and baking mixes), 335 Allerton Avenue, South San Francisco, CA 94080; phone (650) 952-4546, fax (650) 742-6643. Takes orders by mail. Many products will be found in natural food stores and some in grocery stores under "Pamela's" label. Write or phone for their order form.

The Really Great Food Co. (rice and tapioca flours, xanthan gum), PO Box 319, Malverne, NY 11565; phone (800) 593-5377, fax (516) 593-9522. Accepts orders by mail, phone, or fax. Call or write for a product list.

Red River Milling Co. (formerly Sam Pierce Plant) (sorghum, mung, and garbanzo flours), 801 Cumberland Street, Vernon, TX 76384; phone (800) 419-9614 or (940) 553-1211, fax (940) 552-2772. Accepts orders by mail or phone. Products also sold through Miss Roben's and celiac organizations. Company mills only gluten-free products.

Miss Roben's (baking mixes; ready-to-eat products; cookbooks; pastas; a long line of gluten-free flours including sorghum; xanthan gum, guar gum and other baking supplies; plus free technical help and baking support), PO Box 1149, Frederick, MD 21702; phone (800) 891-0083, fax (301) 665-9584, e-mail missroben@msn.com, Accepts orders by mail, phone, e-mail, or fax.

Son's Milling (Romano bean flour and other gluten-free flours), Unit #23, 6809 Kirkpatrick Crescent, Faanichiton, BC V8M 1Z8, Canada; phone (250) 544-1733, fax (604) 389-6719. Accepts orders by phone, mail, or fax. Write or call for complete list. Some products may be found in health food stores.

Specialty Food Shop (mixes, baked goods, pasta, crackers, soups, cook-books, gluten-free flours, xanthan gum, guar gum, rice and corn bran), Radio Centre Plaza, Upper Level, 875 Main Street West, Hamilton, Ontario L8S 4P9, Canada, or 555 University Avenue, Toronto, Ontario, M5G 1X8, Canada; phone (800) SFS-7976 or (905) 528-4707 (Hamilton) or (416) 977-4360 (Toronto), fax (905) 528-5625 (Hamilton) or (416) 977-8394 (Toronto). Takes orders by phone, mail, fax, or e-mail. Write for product list. Also has retail stores in Hamilton and Toronto.

Sterk's Bakery (French bread, dinner rolls, bagels, gluten-free flour, baking mixes, and more), 3866 23 Street, Jordan, Ontario, L0R 1S0, Canada, or 1402 Pine Avenue, Suite 727, Niagara Falls, NY, 14301; phone (905) 562-3086, fax (905) 562-3847. Accepts orders by mail and phone. Write for a free catalog.

Tad Enterprises (rice, potato, and tapioca flours; xanthan and guar gums; bread mix; cereal; pasta), 9356 Pleasant, Tinley Park, IL 60477; phone (800) 438-6153, fax (708) 429-3954. Accepts orders by mail, phone, or fax. Write for order form for complete list of products.

Tamarind Tree (gluten-free shelf-stable, vegetarian, heat-and-serve Indian entrees) 518 Justin Way, Neshanic Station, NJ 08853; phone (908) 369-6300, fax (908) 369-9300. Accepts orders by mail and phone. Products may be found in some health food stores. Check the Web site for a list of products: www.tamtree.com.

This list, offered for the reader's convenience, was updated at the time of publication of this book. I regret I cannot be responsible for later changes in names, addresses, or phone numbers, or for a company's removing some products from its line.

INDEX

Cranberry
   Apple Crisp, 161
   Dressing, 310
   Nut Bread, 79
   Salsa, 311
   Sauce, Spiced, 287
   Walnut Pie, 159
Cream
   Devonshire, 80
   -filled Squash Gems, 78–79
   French, 80
   Rum-flavored Whipped, 180
Creamed
   Cabbage, Old-fashioned, 248
   Chicken à la King, 269
Cream soups, 204–7
   Asparagus, 204
   Base for, 335–36
   Crab or Lobster Bisque, 205
   Curried Tomato, 205
   Easy Chicken, 206
Crescent Crisps, 141–42
Crisp, Cranberry-Apple, 161
Crisps, Cheese, 188
Crumb Topping, 108, 109
Crumpets, 75–76
Crustless Coconut Pie, 158
Crusts, 146
   Absolutely Sinful Cereal, 149
   Almond-Crumb, 117
   Chocolate, 152
   Chocolate Crumb, 115, 116
   Donna Jo's Dream Pastry, 146
   Hash Brown, 260
   Melt-in-the-Mouth Oil, 147
   Mock Graham Cracker, 148
   for pizza, 259
   Ricotta Pastry, 148–49
   Walnut-Crumb, 174
Cucumbers
   Gazpacho, 212
   Icicle Pickles, 253–54
   Sweet Chunk Pickles, 252–53
Curaçao Orange Bundt Cake, 103–4
Curry(ied)
   Beef, with Vegetables, 283
   Cream of Tomato Soup, 205
   Rice, 221
   Rice with Seafood, 221

Shrimp, 324
   South African Fruited, 297
Czechoslovakian Apricot-Almond Bread,
   52–53

Dairy products, 340
   lactose intolerance and, 2–3, 23
Danish (Scandinavian)
   Kringle, 162–63
   Spice Cake with Crumb Topping,
      108–9
Danish (pastry), Fruit, 163–64
Decaffeinated coffee, 9–10
Deep Sea Delight, 325–26
Dermatitis herpetiformis (DH), xviii–
   xx
Desserts, 167–80, 340. See also
   Cakes; Cheesecakes; Cookies;
   Pastries; Pies; Puddings
   African Squash Bread, 78–79
   Almond-Lace Cups, 173
   baked and shaped, 170–73
   Cream-Filled Squash Gems, 78–79
   Down-Under Trifle, 176–77
   Four-Layer, 174
   Light Granola Bars, 190
   Linzertorte, 172
   no-bake, 174–77
   Pam's Pavlova, 170–71
   Pistachio Bars, 175
   Swedish Apple Torte, 171
Devonshire Cream, 80
Dextrin, 10
Diabetics, 23
Dill Dip, Double, 199
Dipping sauces
   Peanut, 200
   Sweet Mustard, 200
   for Tempura, 250
Dips
   Double Dill, 199
   Salmon, 198
   Tartar Sauce, 199
Double Dutch Treat, 111–12
Dough enhancer, 37
Doughnuts
   Baked, 90
   Raised, 89–90
Down-Under Trifle, 176–77

Drop Scones (Scotch Pancakes), 88
Durum flour, 13

Egg(s), 11, 23, 341
  Bread, Jewish (Challah), 54–55
  Crab or Lobster Quiche, 261
  Fu Yung, 262
  Glaze, 139, 140
  Pasta, Fresh, 228–29
  Quiche with Hash Brown Crust, 260
  Replacer Bread, 56–57
Eggplant
  Ratatouille, 241
  Vegetable Parmigiana, 247
Egg Rolls, Chinese, 196–97
English Tea Scones, 80
Entrees. *See also* Casseroles; Luncheon and supper dishes
  Baked Fish Sticks, 318
  Beef Curry with Vegetables, 283
  Cashew Chicken, 306–7
  Chicken in Coconut Sauce, 296
  Coquilles Saint-Jacques, 322
  Corn Soufflé, 245
  Curried Rice with Seafood, 221
  Easy Almond Chicken, 305
  Easy Swiss Steak, 282–83
  Elegant Alaskan Halibut, 316
  Fettuccine with Shrimp and Scallops, 229–30
  Ginger Beef, 284
  Grandma's Chicken Wings, 303
  Haitian Chicken, 300
  Hawaiian Chicken Chunks, 304
  Hungarian Chicken, 299
  Hungarian Goulash, 281–82
  Indian Shrimp Cakes, 323
  Java Beef with Pineapple Sauce, 280–81
  Lentils Marrakesh (with Chicken), 227
  Mediterranean Meatballs, 309
  Moroccan Chicken, 298
  Pork Cutlets with Apple-Brandy Sauce, 286
  Pork with Vegetables, 285
  Scalloped Oysters, 327
  Shrimp Curry, 324

Shrimp-Rice Pot, 321
Singapore Rice Pot, 218
Sole Almondine with Mock Hollandaise Sauce, 319
South African Fruited Curry, 297
Spaghetti Squash Casserole, 246
Stuffed Turkey Rolls, 307–8
Tempura Batter for Seafood, 326–27
Tempura Batter for Vegetables, 249–50
Teriyaki-style Baked Chicken, 301
Tropical Chicken Breasts, 302
Turkey Loaf, 308
Vegetable and Cheese Strata, 244
Vegetable Parmigiana, 247
Envelopes, 10
Eskimo Pie (Ice Cream Bars), 151
Extracts, 10

Fats, 341
Fettuccine with Shrimp and Scallops, 229–30
Fiber, 3, 24
  and Fruit Muffins, 83
Fig and Raisin Filling, Bear Claws with, 164–65
Fillings
  Cherry, 96, 97
  Fig and Raisin, 164–65
  Lemon, 119
  Mock Cherry, 118
  Peanut Butter, 140, 141
Fish, 316–19, 341. *See also* Crab; Shellfish; Shrimp
  Balls, Norwegian, 193–94
  Cake Casserole, Norwegian, 317–18
  Easy Salmon Pâté, 198
  Elegant Alaskan Halibut, 316
  Sole Almondine with Mock Hollandaise Sauce, 319
  Sticks, Baked, 318
  Tempura Batter for, 326–27
Five-Spice Cake, Chinese, 107–8
Flavorings, 10
Flours, gluten-free, 17–22, 331–32, 341
Fool, Rhubarb, 180
Four-Layer Dessert, 174

French
  Bread, Rapid-Rise, 41
  Cream, 80
  fries, 10–11
  Onion Soup, 213
  Ratatouille, 241
Frostings
  Coconut-Pecan, 119
  Mocha Cream, 120–21
Fruit, 341. *See also specific fruits*
  Almond-Lace Dessert Cups for, 173
  Bars, Mediterranean, 134
  Cheesecake Pie, 154–55
  Danish, 163–64
  and Fiber Muffins, 83
  Fresh, Kringle, 163
  Mounds, Christmas, 128
  Sauce, 112, 113
Fruited
  Breakfast Torte, 91
  Curry, South African, 297

Gazpacho, 212
German
  Chocolate Pie, Impossible, 157
  Honey Cakes (Lebkuchen), 139–40
  Potato Patties with Apple and Cheese, 239
GF flour mix, 21–22, 331–32
GF Seasoned Breading, 337
Ginger
  Beef, 284
  Orange Rolls, 76–77
  Rice, 219–20
Gingerbread, 105
Gingers (cookies), Chinese, 136–37
Glazes
  Egg, 139, 140
  Orange, 50, 51
  Orange-Rum, 103, 104
Gluten-free diet, 339–42
Gluten-free products, sources for, 343–47
Glutens
  defined, xviii
  hidden, 8–14
Goulash, Hungarian, 281–82
Graham Cracker(s), Mock, 87
  Crust, 148

Granola
  Bars, Light, 190
  Bread, Swiss, 48–49
  Cookies, 130
  Light, 189–90
Grated Apple Loaf, 81
Greek
  Bean Soup, 209–10
  Gyros Sandwich, 264
  Moussaka, 274–75
Guar gum, 17, 22–23, 37
Gyros Sandwich, 264

Haitian Chicken, 300
Halibut, Elegant Alaskan, 316
Ham
  Butter-Basted Limas with, 226
  Casserole, Savory, 231–32
Hamburgers, 11
Hardtack, Swedish, 85
Hash brown(s), 11
  Crust, 260
Hawaiian
  Chicken Chunks, 304
  Chiffon Cake, 104–5
  Medley, 63
  Pork and Beans, 225
Herb Sourdough, Italian, 71
Hollandaise Sauce, Mock, 319
Honey Cakes, German (Lebkuchen), 139–40
Hors d'oeuvres. *See* Appetizers and hors d'oeuvres
Hospital food, 5–6
Hungarian
  Chicken, 299
  Goulash, 281–82
Hydrolyzed plant protein (HPP), 11
Hydrolyzed vegetable protein (HVP), 11

Ice Cream
  Almond-Lace Dessert Cups for, 173
  Bars (Eskimo Pie), 151
  Cake, 114–15
  Roll, 114
Icicle Pickles, 253–54
Icings
  Baker's Secret, 120
  Lemon, 107, 108

356 / INDEX

Melt-in-the-Mouth Oil Crust, 147
Mixes, time-saving, 329–37
  Buttermilk Pancake, 333
  Creamed Soup Base, 335–36
  GF Seasoned Breading, 337
  Mary G's Biscuit, 334
  Onion Soup, 336
  Triple-Duty Muffin, 332–33
Mocha Cream Frosting, 120–21
Modified food starch, 12
Molded salads
  Soufflé, 250–51
  Two-Tone Vegetable, 251–52
Mole, Meatballs with, 279–80
Monosodium glutamate (MSG), 15
Moroccan
  Chicken, 298
  Lentils Marrakesh (with Chicken), 227
  Spiced Brown Rice, 220
Moussaka, 274–75
Muffins
  Almond-Cheese, 82
  Cream-Filled Squash Gems, 78–79
  Fruit and Fiber, 83
  Kiwi, 84
  Triple-Duty Mix for, 332–33
Mushroom Soup, Cream of, 335
Mustard Sauce, Sweet, 200

Nachos, Potato, 197
Navy Bean Soup, Yankee Style, 210–11
Noodle(s). See also Pasta
  Chicken Soup, Japanese, 214
  Deep Sea Delight, 325–26
Norwegian
  Fish Balls, 193–94
  Fish Cake Casserole, 317–18
Nut-Cranberry Bread, 79
Nut flours, 21
Nutty Pumpkin Treats, 129

Oatmeal
  Bread, Mock, 64
  Cookies (Mock), 127
Oil Crust, Melt-in-the-Mouth, 147
Onion
  Bread, Pink, 66
  Soup, French, 213
  Soup Mix, 336

Orange
  Almond Biscotti, 137–38
  Bundt Cake, Curaçao, 103–4
  Ginger Rolls, 76–77
  Glaze, 50, 51
  Pumpkin Bread, 62
  Raisin Sauce, 288
  Rum Glaze, 103, 104
  Sauce, 122
Oriental. See also Chinese; Japanese
  Easy Almond Chicken, 305
  Ginger Beef, 284
Over-the-counter drugs, 12
Oysters, Scalloped, 327

Pacific Rim Cake, 100
Pancake(s)
  Buttermilk, Mix, 333
  Scotch (Drop Scones), 88
Paradise Drops, 126
Pasta, 228–32, 341
  Chicken-Broccoli Supreme, 232
  Fettuccine with Shrimp and Scal-
    lops, 229–30
  Fresh Egg, 228–29
  Savory Ham Casserole, 231–32
  Touch-of-Irish Casserole, 230–31
Pastries, 143–65. See also Pies
  Bear Claws with Fig and Raisin Fill-
    ing, 164–65
  Cranberry-Apple Crisp, 161
  Danish Kringle, 162–63
  Fresh Fruit Kringle, 163
  Fruit Danish, 163–64
Pastry crusts
  Donna Jo's Dream, 146
  Ricotta, 148–49
Pâté, Easy Salmon, 198
Pavlova, Pam's, 170–71
Peach Clafoutis, 112–13
Peanut Sauce, 200
Peanut butter
  Chocolate Surprise Rounds, 140–
    41
  Filling, 140, 141
  Pie with Chocolate Crust, 152
Pecan(s)
  Coconut Frosting, 119
  Wafers, 185

Peppers
  Gazpacho, 212
  Ratatouille, 241
Pickles, 252–54
  Icicle, 253–54
  Sweet Chunk, 252–53
Pie crusts. *See* Crusts
Pies (dessert), 143–60
  Apple, Imperial, 153
  baked, 153–60
  Caribbean Lime, 155
  Crustless Coconut, 158
  Eskimo (Ice Cream Bars), 151
  Fresh Strawberry, 150
  Fruit Cheesecake, 154–55
  Impossible German Chocolate, 157
  Lemon-Buttermilk, 156
  Peanut Butter, with Chocolate Crust,
    152
  Raspberry-Rhubarb Tart with Ri-
    cotta Crust, 160
  refrigerator or freezer, 150–52
  Walnut-Cranberry, 159
Pies (savory)
  biscuit topping for, 334
  Shepherd's, 277–78
Pineapple
  Hawaiian Medley, 63
  Ricotta Cheesecake, 117
  Sauce, 193
  Sauce, Java Beef with, 280–81
Pink Onion Bread, 66
Pistachio Bars, 175
Pizza, crusts for, 259
Pocket Bread, Arab (Pita Bread), 73–74
Polish Potato Chowder, 208
Popcorn Bread, 67
Pork. *See also* Ham
  and Beans, Hawaiian, 225
  Bette's Special Filled Buns, 265–66
  Cutlets with Apple-Brandy Sauce,
    286
  Russian Cabbage Rolls, 276
  Sâté, 194–96
  with Vegetables, 285
Portuguese Vegetable Soup, 211
Potato(es), 236–40
  Baked Chips, 236
  Baskets, 240

Chowder, Polish, 208
Colcannon, 238
French fries, 10–11
Hash Brown Crust, 260
hash browns, 11
Nachos, 197
Patties with Apple and Cheese, 239
Princess, 237
Shepherd's Pie, 277–78
Potato flour, 20
Potato starch flour, 17, 18, 19
Poultry, 289–311, 341. *See also*
  Chicken; Turkey
Prescriptions, 12
Pretzels, 190–91
Princess Potatoes, 237
Puddings, 177–80
  Apple, 179–80
  Creamy Rice, 177–78
  Rhubarb Fool, 180
  Spicy Bread, 178
Pumpernickel Bread, 44–45
Pumpkin
  Orange Bread, 62
  Treats, Nutty, 129

Quiche
  Crab or Lobster, 261
  with Hash Brown Crust, 260

Ragout, Lucile's Chicken (or Rabbit),
  292
Raisin
  and Fig Filling, Bear Claws with,
    164–65
  Orange Sauce, 288
Raspberry
  Linzertorte, 172
  Rhubarb Tart, with Ricotta Crust,
    160
Ratatouille, 241
Refrigerator pies
  Fresh Strawberry, 150
  Peanut Butter, with Chocolate Crust,
    152
Regency Bars, 132
Restaurants, eating in, 4–5, 10–11
Rhubarb
  Clafoutis, 112–13

Rhubarb *(cont'd)*
  Fool, 180
  Raspberry Tart, with Ricotta Crust,
    160
Rice, 218–24
  Almond Cookies, 136
  Citrus, 219
  Creamy Risotto with Apple and
    Cheese, 223
  Curried, 221
  Curried, with Seafood, 221
  Ginger, 219–20
  glutinous (sticky rice), 15
  Pot, Shrimp, 321
  Pot, Singapore, 218
  Pudding, Creamy, 177–78
  Sherried Chicken with, 295
  Spiced Brown, 220
  Vegetable Risotto with Tofu, 222
Rice bran, 19
Rice Dream Bread, 58–59
Rice flours, 17, 18–19, 36
Rice polish, 19
Rice syrup, 12
Ricotta
  Pastry, 148–49
  Pineapple Cheesecake, 117
Risotto
  Creamy, with Apple and Cheese,
    223
  Vegetable, with Tofu, 222
Rolls (breads), Ginger-Orange, 76–77
Rolls, Sponge (cakes), 113–15
  Ice Cream, 114
  Jelly, 114
  Lemon, 114
Roquefort cheese, 14
Rum
  Balls, 135
  -flavored Whipped Cream, 180
  Orange Glaze, 103, 104
Rusks, Flaky Breakfast, 86
Russian
  Black Bread, 42–43
  Cabbage Rolls, 276
  Kulich, 50–51
Rye
  Bread, Sweet Swedish Mock, 46–47
  Sourdough, Sandra's Mock, 72

Sacher Torte, 110–11
Salads
  Soufflé, 250–51
  Taco, 270
  Two-Tone Molded Vegetable,
    251–52
Salmon
  Dip, 198
  Pâté, Easy, 198
Salsa, Cranberry, 311
Sandwiches, 263–66
  Bette's Special Filled Buns, 265–66
  Crab-Cheese Melt, 263
  Gyros, 264
Sâté
  Beef or Pork, 194–95
  Chicken or Pork, 195–96
Sauces
  Apple-Brandy, 286
  Asparagus, 293
  Chocolate, 111, 112
  Cranberry Salsa, 311
  Cream, 335
  Dipping (for Tempura), 250
  Fruit, 112, 113
  Lemon, 121
  for meat, 287–88
  Mock Hollandaise, 319
  Mole, 279, 280
  Orange, 122
  Orange-Raisin, 288
  Peanut, 200
  Pineapple, 193
  Spiced Cranberry, 287
  Tartar, 199
  Tomato, 254–55
Sausage and Cheese Strata, 268
Savory Ham Casserole, 231–32
Scalloped Oysters, 327
Scallops
  Coquilles Saint-Jacques, 322
  Fettuccine with Shrimp and, 229–30
Scandinavian. *See also* Danish; Nor-
    wegian; Swedish
  Lemon-Buttermilk Pie, 156
  Spice Cake, 106
Scones
  Drop (Scotch Pancakes), 88
  English Tea, 80